D1636872

THE FRUIT CURE

THE
FRUIT CURE

THE STORY OF EXTREME
WELLNESS TURNED SOUR

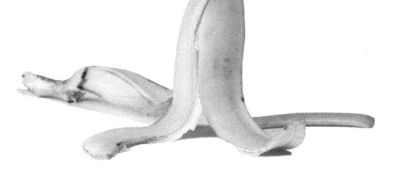

JACQUELINE ALNES

▲ MELVILLE HOUSE
BROOKLYN • LONDON

The Fruit Cure: The Story of Extreme Wellness Turned Sour

First published in 2023 by Melville House
Copyright © 2022 by Jacqueline Alnes
All rights reserved
First Melville House Printing: July 2023

Melville House Publishing
46 John Street
Brooklyn, NY 11201
and
Melville House UK
Suite 2000
16/18 Woodford Road
London E7 0HA

mhpbooks.com
@melvillehouse

ISBN: 978-1-68589-075-9
ISBN: 978-1-68589-076-6 (eBook)

Library of Congress Control Number: 2023944991

Designed by Patrice Sheridan

Printed in the United States of America
1 3 5 7 9 10 8 6 4 2
A catalog record for this book is available from the Library of Congress

To my family, for finding every
possible spot to cheer.

To Eliza, for turning me around.

To Andrew, for the dill pickle chips
and marshmallows at mile 27.

"Beware of false prophets, who come to you in sheep's clothing,
but inwardly are ravenous wolves.
You will know them by their fruits."

MATTHEW 7:15–16

CONTENTS

THE FRUIT CURE

Genesis

BEFORE THE DEFAMATION LAWSUIT, THE CUPS OF COCONUT sugar poured into banana smoothies, the sexual assault allegations, and the dissolution of what was once a dream, there was a man and a woman. Acne covered the woman's face and shoulders and chest. Her gut was inflamed, a symptom of systemic candida. The man, whose father had passed from cancer, was *sick of the lies. Sick of the fries. Sick of rubbing thighs or listening to MLM gurus with dollar$ in their eyes.* And so the man and the woman separated good food from bad. They called the good food Raw, and the bad food they called Murder, Torture, Junk, and Harm.

The man and the woman worshipped what the earth yielded, an abundance of fruits and greens plucked ripe from their vines and stalks and trees. They ate dozens of bananas per day, and mangoes, dragon fruit, persimmons, oranges, peaches, watermelon, papaya, and more. Piles of durian crowned the man's bed. And the woman lay on the ground in a bikini, hair spilling across her face, boxes and boxes of dates surrounding her toned body as the man looked on. The man pressed the fruit between his fingers, saying *squishy, date sugar, nutrition, nutrient-dense*, and neither were ashamed.

The man and the woman held the knowledge of good and evil; they could discern between the sweet flesh of a sun-ripened pineapple and plastic bags filled to the brim with animal blood. They knew that water and carbohydrates in the blood equaled beauty; fat in the blood, ugly. Pure thoughts came from drinking water. With this knowledge, the man and the woman created a website. The man and the woman painted the header with a faded image of browning bananas in the sun. They added green trim to a white background. They added an image of spotty bananas. They renamed themselves Durianrider and Freelee The Banana Girl. With that, the 30 Bananas a Day movement began.

Freelee and Durianrider invited their followers to a fruit farm in Cairns, Australia, where there was a garden and the garden was good. From the garden came tatsoi, a green with leaves like flattened lily pads; Black Russian tomatoes; a bowl of pea-sized cherry tomatoes; tall sprigs of dill; cos lettuce; and sweet leaf skimmed from the stalk. People multiplied, journeying from all around the world. They gathered around a picnic table where the garden's bounty was arranged. Sun overhead, they ate until they were satiated.

Tanned and wiry, the people bore gifts: They whacked a cleaver against a rod of sugarcane before twisting it and twisting it, milking the juice into a bowl. They broke open the scaly green skin of a jackfruit with their fingers. They sifted, smashed, and sieved coconut until it turned to oil, and they slathered it behind their ears, on their shoulders, and into the palms of their hands. They jackhammered avocado, mango, pineapple, and banana in a large pot, poured the golden mixture into a pitcher, drank from it, and said *wow*.

Durianrider, standing before the small crowd of disciples, said, "People just want to feel good." And it was so. There, on the farm, the people slept in tents; the people woke up and ate coconuts; the people went down to the creek for a swim; the people did yoga beneath the limbs of an ancient tree; the people walked the walk and talked the talk and ate raw food and only raw food. *No one snuck down the road for a hamburger.*

Freelee and Durianrider posted footage of toned bodies, testimonies about healing from chronic illness, and images of an abundance of fruit to their site. Through raw food and raw food alone, their followers turned from *flab* to *fab*. From *tragic* to *magic*. From around the world, people watched and saw that the movement was good. Like fruit flies lured by the sweet stench of something overripe, people desperate to heal from eating disorders, to cure illnesses, to save the animals, to find community, and to feel young again were drawn to 30 Bananas a Day.

I was one of them.

CHAPTER 1

The First Fall

A FEW YEARS BEFORE MY FLING WITH FRUIT, I WAS A FRESHMAN in college, a Division I athlete. In the beginning, Coach said, "Run," so I did. I ran eight miles easy, 400 meter repeats, long runs on Sundays, 1200s at a steady clip; I ran anything Coach wanted. I ran through rain, through cold, through illness, and through the ache of too many miles. I ran to meet pain and I ran to escape it. I ran to whittle myself into the number on a clock, faster and faster each time, until Coach said what I had done was good. Even then, I wanted more.

In my wanting, my body betrayed me. One day after practice, I visited our athletic doctor to ask about a cough that had been irritating me for a few weeks. He diagnosed me with bronchitis and gave me a packet of medication to take home. In my dormitory, I took the pills and immediately collapsed. My head hit the wooden leg of a desk chair. When I woke, the objects in my room spun around me as if they belonged in a surrealist painting; the dresser took flight and the white tiles of the ceiling melted into one another.

I blinked. I blinked again, trying to return to the world I had lived in just moments before, but my vision remained warped. My roommate called Coach, who called the doctor, who said my collapse had just been an allergic reaction to the pills; I wasn't to take any of my remaining dose. The doctor said I would be fine in the morning.

The next morning, I woke up with a head that felt full of some atmospheric pressure, as if low clouds had formed. Each time I blinked open my eyes, the ceiling just above my bed blurred before sharpening into focus. I ignored the symptoms. At practice later that afternoon, Coach said, "Run," so I tried. On the track, my team maneuvered like a school of fish: ponytails glimmering in the sun like the flash of scales, each person intimately familiar with the contours of the others. I had been one of them; in many ways, I knew the language of pace and distance better than I knew myself.

But that day, my legs were no longer fluent. The orange of the track spun away from me and the rhythm in my legs felt stilted, out of time. When I angled my body to the track's far curve, I stumbled. My feet hit the interior metal and I fell onto the field. An assistant coach carried me to the training room, where a trainer pressed cool metal to my chest, listened to my heart, and said, "Normal. You are fine." I tried my best to believe her.

On the third day, I lay in bed, dizzy, and Coach permitted me to skip practice but told me I would still be competing in a race two days later. On the fourth day, I boarded a bus even though I was still symptomatic, and on the fifth day, when I woke to the world spinning around me in a hotel room, the doctor's voice in my head said, *You should be fine by the morning.* The memory of the trainer: *Normal.* Months of training with my teammates played like a reel: We had endured freezing rain, hill repetitions, quads so tight they were tender to the touch, barefoot speed sessions across the football field, and the monotony of the same few routes around town. We had made it through bouts of chest colds, the flu, pulled hamstrings, irritated ACLs; we had battled eating disorders and suffered stress fractures. We wore our injuries like medals, using everything we had overcome as evidence of what we could accomplish. Whoever could take the most pain and still compete to Coach's standard was the unspoken winner.

I was reluctant to ask Coach if I could skip the race, which came from a twisted sense of fear and my own eagerness to earn praise through my performance. Coach's role in my life, at that time, was complicated. Her intensity could be beautiful, but mercurial. Sometimes, sitting across from her in her office, I could open up to her about homesickness or running-related anxieties and she would meet me with words of affirmation and her expressive eyes. Her reassurance felt like standing in a thin sliver of sun on a damp day. Had that been her only way of communicating, I probably would have felt comfortable telling her I didn't feel well. But it wasn't. I have memories of her telling us to get our fucking shit together and be fucking heroes or move our fucking asses. She yelled at us after meets when we didn't race to her expectations. She threw her clipboard across the intramural field when we didn't hit our splits. Her anger felt as powerful as her love. I often felt like I was tiptoeing around, trying to please her while harming myself as little as possible. Part of this might have come from the systems in place—during those years, there were fewer public conversations happening about mental health and athletes' wellbeing, and the dearth of female head coaches in the NCAA might have caused the unspoken pressure that she carried—and part of it also came from my own natural tendency to people please, even at the cost of my own health.

Not wanting to disappoint Coach, I got out of bed and made my pre-race oatmeal in the lobby of the hotel. I told myself to toughen up, give the dizziness less power over me. I boarded the bus to the track. I entered the stadium and took a seat on the bleachers. The sounds of my teammates echoed in my ears, and I felt weak, though I had not exerted myself in any meaningful way. When Coach stopped by to check on me, I admitted that I wasn't sure if I could run, let alone race. She sent me to the trainer, who declared me normal. Coach's eyes flashed with what looked to me like annoyance and she said, "Run." So I tried. I followed my teammates outside for a warmup. Flakes of snow drifted toward the ground and the sky was an oppressive kind of white: low to the ground, cloudless. I moved my feet, closing my eyes as often as I could manage. When ten minutes were up, someone opened the door to the indoor track and I stepped inside. The walls became formless, pixelated. And then there was darkness.

When I blinked into light, my head was resting on hard rubber and my legs were propped on a metal chair. Coach stood over me and so did the athletic trainer. The stadium buzzed with the clatter of vaulting poles, and beside me, on the track, I watched the dance of the leaders as they switched positions in the race I was supposed to have run. I listened to the staccato of spikes sticking to rubber, the sound of the crowd that seemed so far away.

*   *   *

After the meet, I visited the athletic doctor, who told me the medication had probably taken just a little longer to work its way out of my system than he initially thought it would. In the days since my first collapse, the symptoms had taken on a rhythm of their own. Oceanic in a way, they flooded in waves before receding. For parts of days, I almost felt like my old self again, capable of talking and walking and seeing. Then, without warning, I would lose control over my limbs and eyes. When my vision became blurry, my head would start rocking back and forth on its own, like an unwilling marionette.

The doctor told me to continue running, so I tried. Day after day, I showed up at afternoon practice and attempted to keep pace with my teammates. Day after day, while in motion, the burnt orange track would melt into the crisscross of the fence and blue of the sky. No matter how many times I tried to blink myself back into the world I had once run through with ease, every formerly familiar marker of geography remained incoherent. Fearing Coach's anger and fueled by the doctor's reassurance that I should be capable of running, I tried letting my legs carry me through the symptoms. Sometimes, I was successful. Othertimes, I would stumble over the metal guardrail or end up in a wide lane, and the assistant coach would carry me to the training room.

The unknowns bothered me the most. How could I be fine for hours while attending class, and then fall on the track? My legs were made for running. No matter what questions I asked, no matter how I tried to push through stuttering steps, my ailment remained invisible. No x-ray to show Coach to prove my limp, no eye test scoring me blurry. Blood tests for West Nile virus, Lyme disease, encephalitis, meningitis, and yellow fever came back clear. I visited an optometrist and a cardiologist at the hospital; both appointments returned no abnormal results. My vitamin levels came back normal, and an on-the-spot reading of my heart returned nothing out of the ordinary. The athletic doctor reiterated that I should be feeling fine. While I'm sure his comments were intended to inspire confidence in me as I attempted to return to running, his reassurance began to feel stale. The chasm between how I felt and how he described me grew wider.

After several appointments, he asked if I would like a referral to a neurologist off-campus. I said yes. A teammate dropped me off at the hospital, and I weaved my way through the maze of halls with aged carpet until I reached neurology, located between a set of bathrooms and gynecology. Alone in the waiting room, I held onto a shred of hope that the doctor might be able to make meaning of my symptoms; I wanted them to be controlled in the same way I could pace myself through a hard set of intervals. When a nurse called my name, I followed her back.

"How are you doin', sweetie?" she asked. She took my height and weight, led me into a room, and took my blood pressure. "That's low, girl." After painting a statistical portrait of me on the intake form, she left the room. She said a doctor would be in soon. I stared at the "What to Do if You Have a Stroke" poster on the wall—call 911, look for drooping of the mouth, ask the person to repeat a phrase, and listen for unintentional repetition or slurring—until I heard a knock on the door.

"The doc at your school called," the doctor said. He half-mumbled, half-sang his words. "He thinks you had a bad reaction to a Z-Pak. Blurry vision. Vertigo. Two episodes of syncope."

"Is syncope fainting?" I asked. I felt as if the language of my body had been translated into something indecipherable. I wanted to snatch it back up, describe the incidents in my own words. The way my head kept rocking back and forth like a distressed animal at the zoo. How my legs wilted from under me like the stems of new flowers.

"Yeah, yeah," he crooned. "You been runnin'?"

"I've been trying," I said. He didn't look at me while he wrote, and I wondered how closely he was listening. "I get really dizzy each time. I usually can't walk well for the rest of the day because my vision gets so blurry."

"Your vision is blurry? How?"

"You know how you can unfocus your eyes on purpose when you're bored in class or tired?" I asked. "Mmm," he mumbled, so I kept talking. "It's like when your eyes glaze over, but you can snap out of it at any moment. With me, I can't snap out of it, no matter how hard I try. Everything around me just stays out of focus."

"Okay," he said. He pulled out a mallet and tapped my knee. My lower leg reacted as it should, swinging forward like a pendulum. "Touch your right hand to your nose, then touch my hand," he said. I did, without difficulty. When he was satisfied, he told me to change hands. I completed the task successfully, and he asked me to follow a pen with my eyes—left, right, left, right—which I completed as well.

"Get up and walk," he said. I walked the two or three steps that it took to get to the door, then back again to my chair. "Looks fine."

"The dizziness comes and goes. Sometimes it gets to the point that

I can't leave my bed. My teammates moved my mattress to the floor because it was getting too difficult for me to climb the ladder," I said, as if the detail would convince him I was telling the truth. I wanted the doctor to know that my symptoms were real. Outdoor Conference, one of the biggest meets of the season, was just a few months away, and I would do anything to be there. I wanted to tell the doctor that sometimes I imagined my legs strong, churning mechanically around the bend of a track, my eyes holding steady to what was ahead.

"Mmm," the doctor mumbled. "Well, I've been in contact with your athletic doctor at the university, and we think you might be suffering from a case of vestibular neuronitis."

"Vestibular . . ."

"It's an inflammation of the vestibulocochlear nerve," he said, and then paused. Keeping his hand on his goatee, he studied the shape of my confusion. "Okay. There's a nerve located in your inner ear that sends information about balance and head position to the brain. When the nerve becomes inflamed—which we believe yours is—the communication between your brain and inner ear is disrupted."

I took notes while he talked. He explained that the symptoms of vestibular neuronitis were usually blurry vision, vertigo, and an inability to balance. Movement becomes a severely botched translation within the language of the body.

"How long will the symptoms stay around?" I asked.

"The most severe symptoms in these cases usually last one to two weeks," he said. I made a mental calculation. Three weeks had passed with symptoms that showed no sign of fading. "There might be some residual issues with balance, but those should be gone within six weeks at most."

"What about running?"

"Now? You technically should be fine," he said. "But if you're feeling symptoms, maybe hold off a week and then ease back into it."

I laughed. "My coach doesn't ease back into anything."

*   *   *

When I think back to those weeks, they are a blur of unread books for class, dizzy walks to the dining hall, hours lying on the cool leather bench of the training room or my mattress on the floor, and the sensation of being hoisted over a teammate's shoulder and carried home. The memory of those days aches with a loss so deep that when I try to return to them, it is as if a fog enshrouds me. The memories aren't memories, but more of an atmosphere.

But the way I remember it isn't entirely true, or maybe I just have a hard time reconciling the two different versions of my body that existed at the time. On one hand, I was succumbing to debilitating symptoms on a regular basis. But my life was also full. My roommate and I had become best friends, and we lived the kind of life that had previously only seemed to exist in movies or my imagination. We played pranks on the boys who lived across the hall, danced in our dorm room to a playlist we had curated, and talked about parallel crushes we had on two of our teammates. We dreamed about becoming team captains as seniors, left each other pick-me-up notes when someone had a tough race or a bad practice, and reminded each other of what we sometimes forgot to see in ourselves: our own strength.

When I got sick, my roommate encouraged me to run—and, because it came from a place of love rather than pressure, I must have tried, even if just for a few weeks. I wish I could say I remember those final training runs, my legs keeping pace with the women around me. But I don't. I have no way of knowing if I felt fear that I would fall or if, at that point, I could still trust the doctor enough to believe that I was capable of recovering. I can imagine during those final miles that I still held hope for what was ahead. After all, that's part of the allure of running. As soon as you hit a split you don't believe you'll be able to manage, you hunger for more. Sometimes in those days, and even still now, I ran as much for the promise of what I believed in as I did the sweet burn of reality.

Perhaps it was that hope for a future self that drew me to the line in late January, just weeks after I had first collapsed. I remember that it snowed that day. We were in Virginia, at Liberty University, and Coach had brought a smaller crew of runners. This meant we got to see her softer side. Instead of telling us we looked like shit-shows or giving us the silent treatment, she brought us to Starbucks and teased us about silly stories we had told on the ride up. I don't remember many details from the meet—not my roommate, not the hotel, not the breakfast I ate, not the warmup—except for the briefest of sensations from my race: The track was a dark rust color and I remember feeling in control of my body. My legs were light and springy, and I lost myself entirely in the motion of the race, those quick laps around the 200-meter track.

When I crossed the line, I realized I had broken my personal 5K record by fifteen seconds. Coach smiled and put her hand on my shoulder. She whispered in a knowing way about how fast I would run later that season in the 10K at Outdoor Conference. I was hopeful. My body had betrayed me, but I had claimed it back.

* * *

After the meet, my symptoms returned. My head would rock back and forth on its own, and I spent hours with my eyes closed in an attempt to quell the sense of discomfort radiating from inside my skull. When I went to a follow-up with the neurologist, he told me that the vestibular neuronitis should have long worked its way out of my system. The doctor on campus echoed him, as did the athletic trainer: "Fine, normal, fine." To hear doctors declare me "fine" day in and day out— and to feel the rough fabric of a blood pressure cuff around my arm, only to hear a trainer declare me "okay"—skewed my ability to listen to my body. Because I was so new to illness, I wanted to believe the medical professionals. I wanted to believe that I was imagining the neuronitis and that I simply wasn't strong enough to push through discomfort; it was easier than convincing myself I was right and the doctors were wrong.

So when Coach said, "Alnes, run the warmup," one day at practice, I listened. On the track, the other girls bunched together at the starting line. They looked at me warily, as if I were a sick animal who might infect the herd. I wasn't wearing my watch. When theirs beeped with the synchronization of a start, I lifted my feet from the ground and followed them. I turned my legs over in their familiar cycle, but I felt far away from myself as I ran. I quickly fell behind the pack. In front of me, the group of runners was a conglomeration of tight abdomens, angles of leg muscle, and hip bones hugged by spandex shorts. I stayed in lane two. Only 200 meters in, my legs tired with effort. My left foot began to pronate inward, as it always did when I was fatigued.

More than anything at that time, I wanted to snap out of my symptoms, or to somehow run through the pain as I had so many other times in my life. In high school, I only missed a few meets for near stress fractures or hip issues. I rarely missed a run. I ran through a bone growing through my big toe, racing with a bloody, open wound for weeks that I refused to get surgery for until I had completed the State meet. In my binder from those years, where I meticulously kept track of my training on hole-punched pages, there are weeks I wrote "windy," "legs hurt," "felt like bricks," and "SLOW," but my weekly mileage totals remained the same, no adjustment made for fatigue or specters of injury. I was praised for my dedication, held on a pedestal for running through shin splints, immense exhaustion, or bouts of seasonal sickness. When other girls on my high school team caved because of the common cold or shortened their runs because of soreness from previous workouts, I convinced myself that I was somehow a better runner because of my unwillingness to do the same. My coach reinforced the idea that running was a mental game; weaknesses of the body were to be overcome.

It is only now that I realize how dangerous that mindset was. My entire self-worth hinged upon my ability to run well; I couldn't conceive of myself in any other capacity. There wasn't room within the sport for recovery, at least not the kind I needed at the time. Running was steeped in measurement: mileage per week, place on the team at each meet, place in the race, splits at practice, length of long runs, how many repetitions of exercises you completed in the weight room, how many times per day you ate, how much you weighed, heart rate, and 5K times. While living within this world of numbers, I found immense satisfaction and value. I could tell if I was doing "well." On the team, anything outside of numbers wasn't necessarily valued. We didn't talk about running holistically, as a sport that might wax and wane throughout life based on a number of factors, like puberty, external emotional stressors, life transitions, or age. We didn't celebrate the chance to run across the intramural fields most mornings, the grass bowing under the weight of pearled drops of dew. We didn't say it was okay for a girl to take six weeks off for injury and wait for her to make a slow but sure return. We wanted results, and we wanted them fast. We wanted splits hit and new personal records.

Running, especially at a Division I school, meant commitment, an expectation that anything happening outside the realm of the track would be ignored as soon as you got there. Girls ran through pain, grief, no sleep, disordered eating, and illness. Because my entire identity was based around the sport, and because I had built my world in college from the foundation of practices, weights, study hall, and friendships on the team, I could not even consider the idea of giving it up. Instead, I told myself that medical professionals had told me I was fine, so I would be.

On the track, the girls ahead of me chatted about classes, the weather, and what they might do in practice later. Their voices sounded far away. I began to feel like I was in an echo chamber, one where the sound of my jagged breaths were repeated back to me. All I could focus on was the shaky sound of *huhhhhhhh-heeeee-huhhhhhh-heeeeeee-uhhhh* emanating from my mouth.

When my roommate looked over her shoulder to ask, *"Are you okay?"* her face was only a blur, her words a cluster of sounds that ricocheted around in my head.

Are .... you ..... okay ...... are ..... you ...... okay? Are you okay?

I couldn't tell if I answered or not. I focused on bringing each of my arms forward and back, forward and back, as if the motion alone would propel me toward the end.

In my old body, the last hundred meters of any workout felt like a homecoming. I remember digging into the grit of myself, pushing my legs through lactic acid, stoking the burn until I thought I couldn't bear it, and crossing the line with decisiveness, as if it were punctuating the end of a sentence. That day, even at a slow pace, each step of the straightaway was uncomfortable. My hips ached. My legs felt like twin boulders, unwieldy. I began a chant of *hate, hate, hate.* I hated myself for not being able to run without failing. Hated the recent memories of afternoons spent in bed, rocking my head back and forth against my pillow, an indentation left behind. Hated remembering the professor who told me that if I could walk, I should be in class—and hated myself for walking there even when I was unable to read or speak. Hated disappointing Coach over and over again. Hated feeling like the doctors were right and I was just weak or scared to get back out there. Hated not knowing when or if I'd ever return to my body as it had been before I first fell.

When I crossed the line, I turned away from Coach. I knew that most likely I looked fine. But something in my head still didn't feel right. When Coach called everyone over, her voice sounded delayed, as if I was in a teeming airport and someone had called my name over the intercom. It took me a moment to hear what she had said, and even longer to respond. She shot me a sharp glance.

"You ladies will be doing thousand-meter repeats today," Coach said. Some of the girls visibly grimaced. "The last few hundred meters should hurt on these, especially as we get to the later intervals."

Coach listed off paces for each group, and the girls took the line. When they'd all flown into their first strides, she asked if I was up for a few easy miles around the track.

"Uh," I hesitated. I wanted to tell her yes. I wanted to run without pause, but I could not ignore the bleariness that tugged at my vision, the way I felt so far removed from my frame. "I don't know if I can."

"Record times then," Coach said. She handed me the clipboard and moved to the inside of the track. Yelled, *"Pick it up!"* to the other runners. I stared down at the list of empty split boxes next to each name. "Alnes" was absent. I bit the inside of my cheek and the names began to dissolve in a teary haze. When I first became ill, the prospect of losing this sport never seemed probable; I could endure anything, I believed. But standing on the side of the track, having not completed a workout in weeks, my name erased from the roster, I wondered about my future. Without running, who was I? I did not want to find out.

*   *   *

There are endless ways to write an origin story. Over the years, I've succumbed to the temptation of rewriting this beginning, as if returning to that first night will give me answers or allow me to change what happened. Instead, holes in the narrative emerge. Why did I keep listening to Coach when she told me to run, even though it resulted in me collapsing on the track? Why didn't I push for answers from the athletic doctor, or make clear to him that the symptoms were not all in my head? Why didn't I call my parents, who I know would have affirmed my symptoms and done anything they could to help me heal?

Looking back now, over a decade later, I want to tell my younger self to get off the track, fly home, and stop running until I have a diagnosis. In theory, I understand why I didn't. At the time, I was a thousand miles away from my family, conditioned to run through pain, and eager to succeed in a sport I deeply loved. Rather than being aware of the fact that my coach and the doctors, as adults in positions of authority, should have been listening to my symptoms and trying their best to protect me, I began to internalize my illness as somehow being my fault. Even after I was admitted to the ER for a night in response to symptoms, and even though I had not been able to run for weeks, I lied to my parents over the phone, telling them I was just taking a few days off because of the bronchitis. Echoing the doctors, who I then believed, I told them I was fine.

Framing my experience this way helps me, to an extent. But as I think now about the darker parts of my story that came after those first few weeks—the ways I tried to harm my own body, the slew of bad cures I reached for in a misinformed attempt to help myself heal—deeper questions plague me. Are the choices I made during those first few weeks of illness the reason that I still to this day have neurological issues, or was it fate? What compelled me to isolate myself from my family when I needed them most? And what, on a psychological level, compelled me to punish my body again and again on the track rather than giving myself permission to rest?

I found answers in a story that resonated with my own, one that unfolded 8,000 miles from here and many years before I first fell ill.

CHAPTER 2

Edenburg

AT THIRTY YEARS OLD, IN 1954, ESTHER (ESSIE) HONIBALL WAS the picture of health: She lived in the city of Pretoria, South Africa, exercised regularly, and worked as a Health and Physical Education lecturer at Pretoria Normal College. She taught classes like Fundamentals of Rhythm, where students choreographed movements to specific beats. The university where she worked was modest but beautiful: The main building on campus was a double-winged structure; a bell tower rose from the center. An avid swimmer and diver throughout her life, Essie walked to campus to swim laps religiously each day. Essie must have loved the feeling of control that came from moving her body through the water—the long, languid motion of muscle, the ache from expended effort afterward. There's a sort of power inherent in crafting the capabilities of your form. Essie's carefully executed dives from the board after laps, which earned her championship titles as a teenager and later as an adult, might have been a comfort, some sort of home.

Thinking about this time in Essie's life—so sweet with promise—feels like remembering my own last days running at the university level. Sometimes when I think back to my last race, though I didn't know then that it would be the last, I want to live in that moment for a while longer. My legs were strong beneath me, and I had no fear of them failing. I want somehow for Essie to stay in the pool, to feel the cool water against her skin, to keep pulling herself forward. In many ways, I wish I could suspend her story here. But instead, as suddenly as my life changed, so did Essie's. Just like mine, it all started with a cough.

Perhaps it was on her walk to school—possibly as she passed the flowering jacaranda trees that bloomed purple and, later in the season, snowed color onto Pretoria's streets—or during a lecture, or while doing research in her office that Essie first coughed. Maybe she thought nothing of it at first—she might have deemed it a result of allergies or a common head cold—but soon the cough gave way to intense and unmistakable symptoms: night sweats, chest pain, and weight loss. She coughed up blood. Essie had developed tuberculosis. Her body, muscular and fit from swimming hundreds of thousands of meters over the course of her lifetime, rapidly grew weak and ravaged by disease. One day, on the pool deck, she searched for a chair where she could lie out in the sun and warm her thinning limbs. She was so weak that she could not lift her feet high enough to clear a garden hose. In her memoir, *I Live on Fruit: Eat more fruit for a fruitful life*, she recalls that a man rushed to her side, saying, "Let me give you a hand, Granny," despite the fact that she was in her early thirties.

Unable to perform her work as a lecturer and too weak to ease her body into the water, Essie admitted herself into a sanitarium, where she hoped to be healed.

*   *   *

A picture of Essie from this time is haunting in the way that her features capture illness; the ridges of her neck cartilage protrude from her gaunt frame; her dark, short hair looks thin; and her eyes are sunken into her face. She tries to smile, but her lips remain close to a straight line.

The sanitarium where Essie was treated no longer exists, but I imagine her lying in bed, the sheets cool against her body while a gentle knock sounds at the door. The doctor who attended to her was brilliant. As someone who was not only invested in her own healing but believed deeply in medical care due to her own work as a health lecturer, Essie gave herself over to the doctor entirely, trusting in his ability to treat her. He put her on medication and told her to rest.

Rest didn't come easily, for several reasons. One is that Essie's doctor entered her room for more than just medical visits. Though he was married, he and Essie engaged in a sexual relationship. Because of Essie's secrecy about this particular time period, there is no way to know whether or not she consented to these interactions or whether she was drawn to the doctor on an emotional level. Essie remained deeply ashamed of this situation for much of her life. Her belief in God contributed to this, as did cultural constructs. As Essie's biographer Anoeschka von Meck explained to me, in South Africa at the time, women who had sex outside of marriage were made to believe they were unworthy of being wed or invited into polite society. At the time, too, Essie was reckoning with the loss of a long-term, codependent relation-ship with another man who had married someone else; she had found out about his marriage only through an announcement in the local newspaper, which further broke her heart.

The second reason for her sleeplessness was that at night, as the weeks passed, Essie began to hear the eerie sound of moths fluttering against the windowpane—hundreds of them. The noise so disturbed her that Essie took to wandering the empty halls of the sanitarium. One of those nights, she opened a closet door where brooms and other miscellaneous items were kept. She found a stray piece of paper and realized it was the label to the medication she had been prescribed. The label told her what the doctor had not: The medication had the poten-tial to destroy her eardrums. The moths she was hearing were not in fact insects, but the sound of her eardrums disintegrating. Unable to leave the sanitarium until her treatment was complete, Essie felt trapped in layers of heartbreak. Not only was she losing her hearing, but her doctor had betrayed her.

Rather than express her grief and anger toward anyone else, Essie unleashed it on her own body.

*   *   *

When Essie was just a child in Edenburg, South Africa, her mother told her to eat the food on the table: bread, eggs, sausage, and jam for breakfast; some combination of steak, mutton, pork, potatoes, pumpkin, squash, and beans for dinner. But Essie refused. Even when her parents promised to buy her a bicycle if she ate meals at home, she ran away to the family's orchard, where she plucked apples from their branches, eating them pip and all. Perhaps her peckish eating habits were somehow innate; between her and her twin, she was always the smaller one. But after being released from the sanitarium, Essie's disinterest in food took a new, perilous tone.

It's not clear whether her relationship with the doctor ended in the sanitarium or after she was out,, but they remained connected by one terrible secret that Essie bore alone: She discovered she was pregnant. Without resources to end the pregnancy, without cultural or social support for unwed pregnant women, and without any hope that the doctor would somehow care for her emotionally, Essie decided she wanted to die. She stopped eating. In a stroke of dark irony, she took up her old job as a lecturer of health and fitness. Too weak to shower or change her clothes, Essie just shuffled home each night, collapsed into bed, and then returned to school in the morning. No matter the weather, Essie donned a heavy coat when she was outside. When she removed her outerwear at school, her students gasped. She was so thin that her formerly fitted clothes looked unnaturally baggy.

Had it not been for her younger sister's upcoming nuptials, there's no way to know what might have happened to Essie. But Essie was asked to be a bridesmaid, and so she went to a dress fitting with a seamstress. When the woman saw Essie's skeletal frame and her skin covered in fine hair, she refused to fit her for a dress. Instead, she gently told Essie that she knew someone who could help her. Essie was so far gone at that point, closer to death than life, that she agreed without argument. The seamstress took her to an addition on the back of a house. Inside the small, spartan room was one chair and a man. The man was not friendly or talkative. He did not greet her with "pleased to meet you" or "hello." The man was Cornelius Valkenberg de Villiers Dreyer, and he offered Essie a cure.

Over twice Essie's age, Cornelius, at seventy-six, lived alone. He devoted time to formulating his "hypothesis," which, simply, was that eating fruit and fruit alone led to optimal health. He made the diet based on no formal nutritional schooling, no scientific evidence, and no formal research, but was curious enough to test its effects on another human. As Essie phrases it in her memoir, "fate probably decreed that when the experiment was ready to be conducted, a suitable human guinea-pig would come to the fore, someone who was prepared to offer herself and submit to relentless discipline." Essie offered herself as just that. On the day of their first meeting, when Cornelius asked Essie to lie down in his room, she did. He moved his hands over her form and determined that she was pregnant, though he kept that a secret from the seamstress who had accompanied Essie to his home. When he was finished with his examination, he asked Essie if she would be his patient. She accepted, but Cornelius and his demands soon brought her closer to death than to any sort of health.

Though the tuberculosis had left her body, Essie continued to experience nausea, skin rashes, insomnia, loss of appetite, and pain. Essie describes herself at the time as "wasting away like a diseased plant." I imagine that her pregnancy was a source of distress, and that her disordered eating clouded her perceptions of what true healthy living and freedom in food might look like. And so, on the first day of the diet, when Cornelius said, "Fast," Essie did. She drank two glasses of distilled water every hour, and though she was unbearably weak, she forced herself out of bed to go to work. On the third day, Cornelius said, *"Eat one piece of fruit every seven hours."* Essie did. She lived on a peach for breakfast, a pear for lunch, and twelve grapes at night.

Those days were hellish for her; she dropped to a weight of sixty-nine pounds. While Cornelius promised Essie relief from her symptoms through his list of rules, she was not immediately healed. Instead, at her low weight, Essie began fainting regularly. She fell flat on her face while getting out of chairs, and it was impossible for her to climb stairs until Cornelius "taught [her] the secret of correct breathing." She experienced other startling symptoms too: Her ears sang, pains reverberated throughout her body, and "cramps made [her] body go rigid from head to toes." As she admits in her memoir, she was clearly a case for hospitalization. Her family and friends expressed their desire to admit her for treatment, but scarred from her experiences in the sanitarium and lured in by Cornelius's promises, Essie refused.

In her memoir, Essie writes that the curative fruit diet devised by Cornelius in 1958 was not only "totally unheard of, both socially and scientifically," but also considered "evil." What Essie didn't know at the time was that both her family's and the public's wariness over the extremism of the fruit cure did hold some validity; Cornelius was hiding dark secrets about his past as a food pioneer that he hoped to take to his grave. His beliefs about food stemmed from a twisted Eden; one steeped in racism, patriarchy, and warped Christianity.

*   *   *

Had Essie flourished immediately on the fruit diet, it might be easier to understand why she stayed with Cornelius. But instead, at her weakest, drinking water as a substitute for meals and longing for the foods "denied to [her]," it is difficult to see why she put all her trust into the commandments of a near stranger. Perhaps, with her grief for her lost body, anxieties about her pregnancy, and her physical weakness, Cornelius's authoritative demands looked like comfort rather than a cause for alarm. Rather than relenting to her family's concerns for her health or recognizing her own severely malnourished body in a capacity that might allow her to escape such rigid eating rules, Essie instead developed an "obsession" with the fruit diet and felt she "had to keep going, at all costs." Her zealotry seemed to echo Cornelius's. His belief in the diet outweighed his compassion for Essie, who was wasting away in front of him. He showed "no mercy to himself and even less" to her.

When I read Essie's memoir, it was difficult to understand why a lecturer of health—someone who could map striations of muscle, who spoke the language of blood and bone—would willingly buy such an absurd prescription for healthfulness. Why would Essie offer herself as a "human guinea pig," even while her family expressed concerns over both her relationship with Cornelius and her rapidly deteriorating weight?

CHAPTER 3

"Well developed female in no acute distress"

A FEW WEEKS AFTER THE NEUROLOGIST TOLD ME MY vestibular neuronitis should be gone, I stood in the doorway of my dormitory. My roommate asked if I wanted to go across the hall to watch a movie with the boys who lived there. I looked back at her and responded, "Do you want . . . do you want . . . do you want?"

She laughed.

I laughed.

She said my name.

I responded, "Jackie, Jackie, Jackie, Jackie," as if I were calling out to myself. Maybe I was. For eighteen years of my life, I had moved through the world feeling sure of my limbs and tongue, but that night, I grew terrified of my own form. Part of me became a ghost. Jackie, Division I runner, disappeared. I knew the words I wanted to say ("Yeah, that sounds fun") but my voice spoke something different ("Jackie, Jackie, Jackie, Jackie"). I stared at my roommate, in hopes my eyes could communicate my fear. My mouth opened and closed like a fish pulled from water.

My roommate told me to stay where I was and ran across the hall to tell the boys. Alone, I tried speaking aloud to myself. *I want to watch a movie*, I thought. But a guttural series of "I, I, I, I" emerged instead. The boys from across the hall, some of them teammates, crowded into the room. I sat down cross-legged on the carpet. The boys loomed over me. My limbs tensed when one of them stepped closer.

"Watch," my roommate said. I felt like an infant, or an animal. "Jackie, can you answer me?"

"Watch," I said. "Watch, Jackie, Jackie, Jackie, hey, hey." My head began to pound. My brain felt like a fist clenched tight.

One boy looked at another. Both of them grinned. "Good one, ladies," one said. "We're gonna go back and play Madden now if this is all you had to show us."

They stood with their arms across their chests and traded looks of disbelief.

"I, I, I, I, I . . ." I said. I wanted to tell them all that I wasn't lying or joking around. My head hurt worse than ever, but nothing of meaning took shape on my tongue.

"She just started doing this before I came to get you guys," my roommate said. I looked at her, hoping she would recognize something in my eyes that would tell her I was trapped. After spending every day together for months, she knew me better than anyone. I wanted her to send the boys away, to call Coach, to tell me it would be okay. I didn't know why the boys were there. Maybe my roommate needed a witness while I morphed into something incomprehensible before her.

"Real funny, guys," one of the boys said. "Now can we go?"

I smiled. I started laughing. Faking an illness seemed preposterous. Once I began laughing, I could not stop. The sound coming from me was maniacal, rising to a shriek in pitch. The boys took it as proof that I was joking. Everyone except my roommate left. I started sobbing. My face felt like a mask I had no control over.

"I, I, I, I . . ."

Once safely in bed, my roommate pulled the covers over me and laid down next to me, whispering *shhh* until the sobs ceased. She murmured me into a light sleep and turned out the light before leaving the room. I pulled the covers over my head and attempted to whisper the words in my head, with no success.

* * *

I don't remember how it started—if I asked, or if my teammates made the decision—but a day or two later, when I experienced another word-finding episode, someone filmed it. I don't have access to the clip anymore, but I remember it being brief enough that someone from my team sent it to my phone, and I brought it with me when I visited the neurologist a few days later. When he walked in, he asked how I was doing.

"Amazing!" I said. I laughed. I wanted to meet his expectations of normalcy. He offered me a polite smile and waited for me to continue. "The neuronitis is leaving my body!"

"You're not experiencing dizziness or blurred vision anymore?"

"Well, yeah, I am, but I think it's leaving because I'm having speech problems," I said. My explanation to the doctor now seems preposterous. I want to sit next to the girl in the doctor's office and tell her to push for testing. Sleep more. Learn to accept that this will be a part of her life. But the girl in the office was in denial. To acknowledge the speech issues as alarming would have been to accept that she might be a patient instead of Jackie.

"What kind of speech problems are we talking about?" he asked.

"I was in my room, and my roommate said my name," I began to explain. "I repeated it back without meaning to."

"You repeated it?"

"Yeah," I said. I felt dumb relaying the events. Based on our previous interactions, I had thought I would come to the doctor, tell him I was on the mend, and that he would be happy to hear it. If he hadn't believed my prior symptoms to be anything outside of vestibular neuronitis, then why would he pursue more details about this?

"I repeated my name. I said, 'Jackie, Jackie, Jackie,' and I couldn't really stop."

"Were you conscious?"

"Yes," I said, hesitating. I had been conscious, but the second episode—the one recorded on video—I didn't remember. I had woken up in my bed with a headache afterward. "I think. I don't remember exactly."

The doctor leaned back in his chair. "You have blurry vision, vertigo, syncope, and now you can't speak. Am I getting this right?"

His words were clipped, which made it seem as though my particular combination of ailments was improbable. I felt like my life and symptoms had become the subject of a trial. Looking back at his notes, it's striking how my lived experience was translated into information that was not deemed credible: "She apparently sat down" or "She denies problems with self-esteem." I remember the brusque line of questioning that occurred each visit.

"Did you really faint?"

"You've had no sexual intercourse? Are you sure?"

"You experienced both aphasia and dizziness? Those symptoms usually don't pair with one another."

"Are you stressed about school? We have other resources, like counseling."

Once, after reassuring the neurologist that I had never had sex, I was tested for pregnancy three times within the span of a week. None of the nurses believed my testimony, and one of them told me, "Girls like you are the reason we have to be so careful."

When I look back at the initial doctor's notes all these years later, I find gaps between my own physical experiences and what was recorded on official documents. These reports have since been passed along to other neurologists and specialists, meaning that other professionals read the neurologist's impressions of me before I have the chance to tell my own story. In a way, the truest story, or at least the most accurate version of my lived experience, has been undercut by phrasing that incites doubt in the mind of the reader and, like most medical documents, reduces me from a person with emotions, hopes, dreams, and a history, to a series of categories and brief tests. I know that this is not my initial neurologist's fault alone. I am sure medical students are taught to scan for certain signs and record information that can be translated from hospital to hospital. But pain and symptoms are tricky; diseases manifest differently from person to person. Why reach for doubt as a first response? What would happen if, instead of putting people into boxes and hoping they meet the exact definition of an illness, the doctor recorded their experiences with empathy instead? With a more holistic view of the patient? I wonder how my story might have changed had my doctor—or Coach or trainer—trusted me, especially during those first impressionable weeks of illness.

In the doctor's office, as an eighteen-year-old, I did not yet know to ask the neurologist what his notes said or think to request my records when I left the practice each visit. Because of his repeated iteration that I should be fine and I should return to normal activity, I was afraid to explain my speech symptoms, which I'm sure influenced his reading of my case as well. Complicating matters was the fact that I appeared completely fine whenever I visited. I never experienced an episode in his office. Knowing all this, I pulled my phone from my purse midway through our appointment, as if offering evidence to a reluctant judge.

"My teammates took this," I said, and hit play. He leaned over to peer at the screen. My voice, warbled and stuttering, emerged tinny from the speakers. After watching, he took notes on his computer. The keys clacked under his fingertips.

"We're going to have to run some tests."

He looked directly at me, brown eyes concerned. I started to grow uneasy, as if I had confessed something that would get me in trouble. The shift that happened within him between my verbal portrayal of events and the video was stark. I wanted to ask him if I'd be able to run Outdoor Conference in a couple of months, but he started to speak.

"This isn't good," he said. "No driving–"

"I don't even have a car!" I laughed, as if the fact that I didn't have a car negated the idea that my physical body could not be trusted to drive. *You are a Division I athlete. You are a straight-A student. Your medical tests are all normal. You are fine.*

"No driving, no physical activity, and get plenty of sleep," he said. "Record these episodes because we'll need them down the line."

I cringed. The words "down the line" made me uncomfortable. I needed to run. "Okay," I managed.

"I'm scheduling you for an emergency EEG," he said.

"Why are we doing this? Isn't this the neuronitis taking a weird turn?"

"Based on what you've told me, it's possible you might be experiencing complex partial seizures." He scanned the monitor as if it were a map. "If I'm interpreting your symptoms correctly, I think that the seizures might be occurring in the left temporal lobe of your brain, the region that controls language comprehension."

"Isn't this part of the neuronitis?" I asked again, pleading. *Let me run the 10K at Outdoor Conference. Tell me my words are mine.*

"No," he said. "We're dealing with something more complicated here."

*   *   *

When I think of Essie, who fervently believed in the fruit cure despite the pain it caused her, I am struck by the trust she put in her doctor at the sanitarium. I think about how lonely it must have been to wake up in her apartment after she was discharged, no one visiting her at night, and even the sounds of the phantom moths gone quiet. I think about how she might have longed for the water of the pool to remind her of the body she had lost. I think about these things because I know too well how the treatment of illness can cause more pain than the symptoms themselves, how thin the line is between care and harm.

The emergency EEG showed no sign of seizure activity, so the neurologist suggested that we monitor symptoms and check back in at a follow-up appointment. Rather than fading away, my episodes got scarier. I continued experiencing symptoms of blurred vision and dizziness (my head would rock in circles on its own, like someone unwillingly participating in a group exercise class) and my speech problems persisted. I shouted things like, "Hey! It's Tim! Hey! It's Tim! Hey! It's Tim!" "Sky news, sky news, sky news," or "Aurora, Aurora, Aurora." Both a balm and most terrifying of all, I began to lose my memory of these events. During the first few episodes, aside from the brief moments I had blacked out, I remembered every symptom and sensation, but I had begun to wake up from episodes without knowing what had happened to me. I would wake up on my mattress, one time clutching a roll of Ritz crackers, sometimes with a sense of fear, and take note—of the pink rug, the cheap wood of the dresser, and the white tiles of the ceiling—as if to remind myself where I was. My own life in those moments became a mystery I couldn't solve.

At the start of my illness, my teammates carried me across campus, let me lean on their shoulders, drove me to appointments, stroked my forehead when I was confined to bed, and promised that I would be back out on the track soon. But after I began experiencing my word-finding episodes, their care turned playful—and then cruel. While I don't remember their actions in a way that allows me to pull each memory from an archive in my mind, my body holds clues of what happened. Even now, over a decade later, if someone tries to hold me during an episode, I resist or scream, even if I deeply trust them. There is some primal sense of fear that I will be harmed while I am vulnerable. This feeling doesn't come from nowhere; the nightmare has already happened.

The cruelty started as a warped kind of care, or at least I interpreted it that way at the time. While I was episodic, my teammates told me to sing, "We are the three best friends that anyone could have," and I did. They handed me sweaters and yelled at me to put one on and then another one and another until I woke up on my mattress, clammy and disoriented, not understanding why I had so many clothes on. My teammates lied and told me my dog had died; they took pictures of me crying and cradling a foam roller and showed them to me the following morning. They told me there were spiders on my back, told me to strip off my shirt, and watched and laughed as I ran down the hall in my bra. My teammates made a bet that one of the boys couldn't kiss me before spring break, and he came in late one night, reeking of beer, pinned my arms to my mattress on the floor while I whispered *no*, and pressed his lips against mine again and again until he fell asleep, his weight pressing me down. I slithered out from under him. Not trusting my legs to carry me past the doorway of my own bedroom and not wanting to wake my roommate, who had a crush on him, I slept on a corner of the rug.

My teammates took another video of me, though this time not for the doctor. In the footage, I'm standing in the doorway to my dorm. I'm wearing black running shorts, a maroon shirt, and brown-framed glasses. The door behind me is covered in wrapping paper, pink and red and white Valentine's hearts patterned in parallel lines. A coloring book page of a frog with a crown says "Kiss Me" and is tacked over the wrapping paper. My face looks round. My eyes have a glossy appearance, and my mouth remains in a smile for most of the footage. At the beginning of the video, I hold my hands against my stomach while I laugh, then grip the doorframe for balance. Behind the camera are my teammates.

MALE 1: Can you talk to us for just a second? Talk to us, Jackie.
ME: I . . . um . . .
MALE 2: What are you doing tomorrow?
ME: I . . . am going to teaching-ing tomorrow.
MALE 1: You mean yesterday?
ME: (Still gripping doorframe, I pause to look down and close my
    eyes before speaking) I . . . I . . . I. (Look at watch.)
    (Laughter.)
MALE 1: Yes, you mean yesterday.
ME: Yeah, yeah, I . . . I . . . I went yes–yesterday. (Laughter from
    two males and one female behind the camera. I laugh
    as well, still holding onto the doorframe.)
MALE 1: You're going yesterday, right?
MALE 2: You went today?
ME: N-no . . . I . . . no . . . I . . . went . . . I went. (Laughter from
    everyone behind the camera. I respond with laughter.)
    I . . . went yesterday! And I'm going tomorrow.
MALE 1: You mean going yesterday and you went tomorrow!
ME: (Stares at camera, smiling, but obviously confused. Still stands
    in doorway, alone.) OW! NOOO!
MALE 2: But you used to go today.
ME: No! Noo! I–no! I–no! I, I. (Camera comes closer to my face,
    revealing me smiling, while still confused.) I went
    to the–
(Everyone behind the camera laughs loudly. I laugh.)
ME: I went to cla–ass.

(More laughter from everyone behind the camera.)

MALE 2: Wait, so, you had to go tomorrow but you went yesterday?

ME: No, no... no, no. (Eyes look up toward the right side of the ceiling.) I went . . . I'm, I'm, I'm went, I'm went.

(Everyone behind the camera laughs loudly.)

FEMALE 1: You guys are so mean. (Laughs.)

ME: I am, I, I. (People behind the camera are hysterical with laughter. My voice elevates to a higher pitch and increases in volume.) I . . . I . . . went yes–terday.

(Loud fits of laughter from everyone behind the camera. I laugh, but my voice sounds distressed.)

MALE 1: Oh, my God. So you went tomorrow?

ME: (Voice is shaky, high-pitched, loud.) No, I, I . . . (I bend my arms and hold my hands up in frustration.) I . . . I . . .

MALE 2: She's gonna cry.

ME: I, I, I, I am, I am . . . I am . . . I am going.

FEMALE: All right, guys, you're stressing her out now.

ME: I, I, I am go–ing tomorrow.

MALE 2: Wait, you're going yesterday and you have gone tomorrow but you will go today?

ME: (Screaming in a high-pitched, broken voice.) I went yesterday. (I laugh.) Yes–terdayyy. I will go tomorrow.

MALE 1: I can't even laugh anymore; my cheeks hurt. Hey, this camera better be on because this is going straight to my computer.

The video was uploaded to YouTube by a member of my team, and I remember watching it the following morning. I laughed. I laughed at everything in those days. I laughed when a teammate called me a whale because I'd grown softer without daily miles. I laughed when one of my teammates said, "You're faking all of this, you freak." I laughed when I was coherent and my teammates rehashed whatever

I had done the night before: I hid under a desk, I repeated the same song for thirty minutes, I cried, I repeated a teammate's name, I looked drunk while trying to walk home from the dining hall and a group of sorority girls stared at me. I laughed and laughed and laughed. None of it was funny, but laughter was a way of pretending I still belonged to the team. If I could laugh with my teammates at the version of myself who was sick, I believed that I could erase her from my own body. If I laughed, I could keep my friends. If I laughed, I might be able to turn everything—all those doctor visits, those unremembered days, the pain of feeling so disoriented in a body that had once responded to every demand—into one big joke, something I could pretend had been a misunderstanding.

*   *   *

Despite the fact that no seizure activity had been confirmed on the emergency EEG, the neurologist put me on seizure medication the next time I saw him. As he explained it, at eighteen, my brain was still malleable. The seizure meds might correct whatever neurons were misfiring so that I would not have episodes the rest of my life. After the first medicine left me with welts the size of golf balls, I was put on a different pill. It gave my days a muted quality, like being underwater. I was underwater when I said goodbye to my teammates and Coach for the summer, boarded a plane, and returned to my family in Missouri, where they looked at me with too-wide eyes when I landed. I was underwater when I left the house to do my runs and found myself frozen in fear. Too terrified of collapsing to try on my own, I walked to the edge of the lake and sat there for the time my daily miles would have taken before heading home. I was underwater when I became episodic at home, and my brother, an EMT, took my pulse, my heart rate, and asked me to remember three words before telling my mom, *"I can't tell what's wrong"*—at seventeen, he knew to do only so much for a body that was failing. I was underwater when I returned to campus, moved into an apartment, and pretended to be Jackie again, that girl who laughed at everything and ran through pain.

I wasn't Jackie anymore. At our annual pre-season camp at a lake house, I went for a run with teammates but found my vision fading on the way back. I tried to keep running through my symptoms, like I had the previous semester. The pine trees lining the road blurred away. I wheezed with effort. I closed my eyes and told myself to put one foot down, and then the other, and keep going straight. The world grew hushed. Coach's voice cut through. "Get in the van, Alnes," she snapped. There was disappointment in her voice, or fatigue. She veered the van toward my side of the road and I stumbled in. I longed for a moment of her softness, for her to call me "buddy" like she had when she sat with me all night in the ER, but that day she was silent. She pressed hard on the gas pedal and tried to catch up to the fast pack. That ride felt like the end of a long relationship; maybe both of us knew it was over, but I wouldn't say it officially until weeks later, in her office, where I would cry and apologize and she would ask me to return my uniform. I would say goodbye to my teammates on the track and we would cry for something that had been lost long before that moment, and then I would walk away on my own.

As strange as this is to remember or confess, until I left the team, I had never really come to terms in any meaningful way with the fact that I might be ill. My whole life had been built around an ability to ignore pain, to play mind games until I made it one more mile or ran just a little bit faster. It was a game I had been playing since middle school. No coach or anyone of authority had ever told me to rest, to acknowledge the limits of my body, or to honor the strength in my legs by also taking it easy. Because so many months had passed with doctors and Coach dismissing my symptoms as being ones I could run through, I had a twisted sense of my own perception of the world.

Was my illness real, or was I somehow faking the whole thing, caving to some phantom voice who wanted me to be weak? What pain was worth stopping for?

In the first days after leaving the team, I felt like some essential rhythm had been lost. There was no early-morning practice, no mid-morning weights, no rush to the shower before class, no looking forward to a pasta party on Friday night at the older girls' place, no race to train for, no times on a clipboard to remind me I was succeeding. Instead, there was stillness. Life without the team was waking up alone in my new apartment, slipping on an outfit I thought Coach would most likely call a shit-show (tie-dye and non-matching athletic shorts). It was sitting alone in the back of every classroom I entered, afraid to speak in case garbled sounds emerged from my mouth. It was hating my voice when I could say my name (had any of the past semester been real?) and hating that my legs never weakened on my walk home. It was going for my first run alone, leaving clear instructions for my new roommate, Eliza, of where I would be and whom she should call if I didn't come home, and taking my first easy steps as an unattached runner. It was making it through three miles and feeling rage that my legs had carried me without a problem, that my vision had remained clear. Months of Coach and the athletic doctor and my teammates telling me to run, and now I could. I was furious.

A grief of seismic proportions—for my lost body, for the girl who had been pressed to a mattress by someone she thought was a friend, for the loss of life without a team, for the laughter, all the laughter, over my stuttering voice—began to break through. I had no idea how to contain it. And maybe, only because the pain was too overwhelming, I couldn't. In the shower one night, I held a razor to my wrist and pressed down. The pain was a small, sharp bite. There was blood, and I felt some relief. I had been submerged for so long that the cut felt like a quick gasp of air. The pain of memory was briefly interrupted by the pinch of metal against skin. I wanted more.

In the following few days, I unraveled with abandon. I wanted to erase the ghost of Jackie, whose pain I carried, who followed me everywhere—to class, where I now introduced myself as Jacqueline; in chance encounters with teammates, during which time I'd politely smile and say I was feeling well; on my stupid daily runs that carried me nowhere near the distance I used to pursue. And for what purpose? What was the point of any of it? I biked to JCPenney and paid fifteen dollars to cut my hair to my ears, straight and blunt all the way around, and then I cut myself on my upper arm that night because I hated what I had done to myself. I wanted a physical pain that could sweep me away from the hauntings of memory for longer than just a moment, and so one night, I tried to lose myself in a way that couldn't easily be undone.

When I remember now what happened, I look at my old self from an aerial view, as if I am forever watching over the girl who left her bed in the middle of the night. Outside, the air is still and calm. Streetlamps wash the road orange. The girl leaves her apartment, runs down the streets she once did with the team. She waits for the act of running to buoy her to some old version of herself, but she feels nothing. No joy, no splits to mark her worth, no team jostling around her. She wheels her legs as fast as they can churn, hoping for some spark of an old life to rekindle, but the effort leaves her winded, lungs searing. Nothing more. The train tracks in sight, she stops. With care, she removes her shoes and socks and shirt. She drapes them over the limbs of a tree before darting out into the middle of the empty road. Stray fragments of asphalt press into the soft parts of her feet. Unlike running barefoot across the grassy field with the team in the past, this night, she seeks pain.

Watch the girl run down the train tracks, only the moon's glow illuminating her path along the corridor of pines. The girl glances left and right in search of a train's light. Taste of copper in her mouth, some urgent beat rapping at the taut drum of her heart. When only silence answers, she tears onto the road. Dancing on the double yellow line, she grinds her heels into the pavement, hoping for blood. When she fails, she runs home to her apartment. Watch as she punches her left wrist with her right fist. Watch as she slams her forearm over and over again against the bathroom doorframe. No bruises blooming on her arms, no desire to be tender toward a body that she believes has failed her, she falls into bed and relinquishes herself to uneasy sleep.

CHAPTER 4

Fleshless, Bloodless, and Poison-Free

IN HER MEMOIR, ESSIE WRITES THAT "[N]O RESISTANCE, OF whatever kind, would have stopped [Cornelius]" from conducting his fruit experiment. In many ways, more sinister than she knew, Essie was right. As Cornelius commanded her to fast, and as he watched her grow weaker and weaker, I wonder if the past and present collapsed until time and place were indistinguishable. Part of him might have been in South Africa with Essie, who grew frailer by the day, while the other half was submerged in memories of Melbourne, where decades before, he had opened a facility called the Valkenberg Naturopathic Hospital and supervised people he called his "patients." There, in a haunting echo of his work with Essie, he had tried to cure a range of ailments—epilepsy, spine troubles, and diabetes—by forcing people to drink only hot water for extended periods of time.

He had come to the field of medicine, if what he performed can in any way be called "medicine," in a roundabout way. The second of six sons born to Melt van der Spuy Dreyer and Maria Elizabeth de Villiers, Cornelius was raised near Cape Town. He played football and tennis, and later claimed that as a teenager he could lift 103 pounds above his head with one hand. In 1901, when he was around nineteen, his father died of Bright's disease and a dropsical condition (in today's terms: kidney inflammation and congestive heart failure), despite the efforts of the best specialists in Cape Town.

While Cornelius attended the National College in Cape Town and worked as an accountant for the Bank of Africa after graduation, he patched together his own medical "studies" of sorts, on the side. Reeling from the loss of his father, Cornelius took inspiration from his elder brother Thomas, who was a medical student at the United Friedrich University (now known as Martin Luther University) in Germany. "I studied text-books with my brother," Cornelius said. "During that time I had plenty of spare occasions to prosecute my studies into the causes of disease. I began to practice on myself and obtained temporary benefits. I prescribed for some of my sick friends." He soon realized that a life of numbers would not satisfy him, resigned from his position at the bank, and traveled to Australia in 1911. He started going by "Robert de Villiers Dreyer"—whether that was to buffer himself legally from Cornelius or just a preference is unclear. In 1916, at the age of thirty-two, Cornelius joined the Australian Imperial Force (AIF). He fought in the Great War (better known today as World War I). Handwritten records from a visit to a doctor in 1917 describe him as having a "moderate ability" and that Cornelius "asked to resign," but his request was apparently denied, as a newspaper article from 1918 mentions that "Cpl. [Corporal] Robert Devilliers Dreyer, South Africa" was wounded ("second occasion"). AIF records show he returned to Australia in 1919. He purchased 334 acres of land south of Perth, near North Dandalup, but later left for Melbourne, where his efforts to heal himself and others ramped up significantly. He began publishing a newspaper and, in a moment that was probably significant to him because of his history with his father, claimed to have "cured a clergyman of Bright's disease." During this time, he was radicalized to believe deeply in the idea that the body needed to be purified from "sin." He believed not only in testing questionable methods of healing himself but viewed it as his mission to save others from illness, too.

One such man was Herman Carl Arnold, who, in 1931, was fifty-five years old and a salesman. His stomach was in great pain. Worried he might have a growth, he paid for an x-ray, which came back negative. He saw a series of specialists, but his pain remained. On September 20, he consulted with Cornelius at Valkenberg Naturopathic Hospital. If Cornelius's book *The Bible of Nature and the Book of Wisdom* is any indication of his methods, Cornelius most likely asked Arnold to lie down so he could lay his hands passively on the cold part of the patient's body. Through his hands, Cornelius would communicate with cosmic forces, which would enable him to alleviate pain without drugs and inform him of the cause of Arnold's illness. In this case, Cornelius deduced that Arnold had something wrong with his spine. Nature could heal him, but it would require a massage and a hot water fast.

On the patient's second day at the hospital, his wife, Elizabeth Arnold, came to visit. Her husband asked for food several times, so she returned with his favorite snacks: biscuits, raisins, marmalade, and nuts. Cornelius made her take them home, saying it wouldn't be right for Arnold to have them. Subsisting on hot water, Arnold grew weaker and weaker. He began to look emaciated and continued asking for food. The only nurse on duty, Violet Caroline Pieta—who had no schooling for the role but had left her waitressing job to be trained in medicine by Cornelius—testified that the patient complained of pains in his right side. Following Cornelius's direction, a week or so into his stay she fed Arnold small portions of cooked vegetables, broth, grape juice, an orange-colored drink, and peanut butter. It was not enough. On October 12, Arnold needed to be propped up by pillows in bed in order to remain somewhat upright. On October 13, Cornelius called Elizabeth to tell her that her husband had a growth in his liver and would need to leave the facility immediately. When Elizabeth arrived at her husband's bedside later that day, he was already unconscious.

"He is dying," she said, but Cornelius told her he was only sleeping. Arnold died at 3:00 p.m. on October 14, 1931. At trial in November of that year, the coroner revealed that there was no growth in Arnold's liver. He did have a small cancerous growth in his stomach, but it would not have killed him for months. He had died from lack of nourishment.

Arnold was not the first man who had died in Cornelius's care. Months earlier, in March 1931, another suit against Cornelius had been filed for the death of a sixty-year-old investor, Arthur Haughton Russell, who had died two days after being released from the Valkenberg Naturopathic Hospital. Russell, a diabetic, had been advised to abstain from taking insulin. He was put on a hot water fast for seven days. Edna Brown, a seamstress prior to enrolling herself as a nurse-in-training at Cornelius's hospital, testified that Russell asked for food often, but he was only given orange juice. The morning of February 23, two days into his stay, his son came to visit and found his father to be all right except for a touch of heartburn, but by nightfall his father was too weak to speak. Russell was taken to a hospital, but by then it was too late. He died because his insulin was cut off at the Valkenberg Naturopathic Hospital.

Others, if confronted with the deaths of two men in their care, might have stopped practicing medicine completely, or at the very least looked into studying the profession in a more structured capacity. (On trial, when asked if he had "taken any course of training" in regard to medicine, Cornelius responded that "practical experience on myself goes further." He explained that he deliberately contracted venereal diseases "not by impropriety," and cured himself as supposed proof of the effectiveness of his methods.) In what appear to be his booking photos taken in February 1932, Cornelius looks directly at the camera with doleful, dark eyes. Standing next to the height chart, he looks almost like a child, not because of his stature but because of the resigned slope of his shoulders and the way his suit, both pants and jacket, are thoroughly wrinkled.

After he was released from a six-month stint in prison, Cornelius took to the streets. In 1933, he preached about his "false imprisonment" to a crowded hall of 300 to 400 people. A detective characterized him as "very nervous at the commencement, later developing into a very forceful speaker with a strong personality." His speech was rambling; he covered everything from "'Wisdom' of the Magic Key" to the economic system and made a gaffe in publicly berating the Ten Commandments, before ending with the claim that he had been tricked by other doctors, which had led to the two patients dying in his care. The detective concluded the report by saying, "It would seem that he is working alone, and that he is definitely 'touched' if not a meglo-maniac, although he has marvellous self-control. He had a strong hold over the audience, demonstrating his hypnotic powers."

His ability to charm an audience apparently won over a woman named Elva Mary Willing, who, though trained as a nurse, became "a convert" to Cornelius's "public teaching." She fell in love with Cornelius's way of seeing the world, married him, then "prepared herself to become a mother of a baby which should prove to the world that human immunity from disease can be attained." (What she did to prepare is not specified.) In 1936, Elva Mary had what the couple deemed "the most vigorous, mentally alert, well developed and healthy baby in the world." They named him Mazda. Though Mazda was declared by newspaper headlines and Cornelius to be the "world's most perfect baby," Cornelius soon found fault in the way that Mazda had been born, namely that the Wahroonga Sanitarium had subjected Elva Mary to "certain X-ray processes unnecessary in the circumstances," which had caused "great bodily harm and pain for a long period." In a pamphlet he published for the public, Cornelius wrote that he expected better of Wahroonga Sanitarium than "baby damnation." On September 28, 1936, it was reported that Cornelius made a claim on behalf of Mazda for "£2000 against the Australian Conference Association Ltd." for "wrongful treatment and conduct." Elva Mary filed a claim for £1,000. She claimed that the doctor in charge said to her, "in a dictatory, emphatic and imperious manner, 'You must drink cow's milk or how are you going to breastfeed your baby? You will have no milk for your child. It won't be able to make teeth and you will lose it.'"

The details of Elva Mary's delivery and the ensuing legal claims aren't necessarily the point. Instead, this and other moments in Cornelius's public life indicate how deeply he had come to believe in his own teachings, enough to disregard the law and permanently alter the course of other people's lives. In his mind—and subsequently Elva Mary's, after converting to his way of thinking—cow's milk was a toxin. In his book, *The Bible of Nature and the Book of Wisdom*, he writes that when he saw people drinking milk, "I could weep like Jesus for the destiny of mankind."

His book offers the most saturated look into his beliefs, featuring entries in the index like "Wholesale Murder," "Puberty and Moon," "Serving the Devil," and "The Salvation Diet," as well as an all-caps section, "MISCELLANEOUS ITEMS FOR UNDERSTANDING TO PROMOTE WISDOM THROUGH TRUE KNOWLEDGE OF THE ARTIFICIAL WORLD." The prologue features a picture of Cornelius's face. In it, his thin lips are pursed, the angles of his square jawline are highlighted by shadow, and his eyes seem to stare beyond the camera. He wants readers to look at him, to make "some sort of judgment of the Author's health," as the more "poisons" you were loaded up with, the "uglier" you got. He believed that if you were ill, it was a sign that you had transgressed and consumed too many "popular toxins." He believed that if you died ill and in pain, you deserved it; you had sinned. He equated "natural food" with moral goodness ("A natural man is a healthy man, and a healthy man is a moral man") and insisted that if boys were allowed to partake in any food but what was "natural," they would cock their ears for "smutty yarn" and steal "clandestine glances at the legs and shaking breasts of the flapper." (He was, as an adult man, also particularly concerned for "little trustful girls," the "freshness" of "infantile" nineteen-year-olds, and the constipation he insisted that "more than ninety percent of girls suffer.")

Most surprising of all, considering his later experiment with Essie, in the 1930s, Cornelius believed that fruit was a fallacy. "Fruitarians and other food faddists ascribe to fruit a health-giving potency which is entirely erroneous," he writes. "Fruit is not essential to health." He also discloses that Elva Mary developed anal fissures after eating fruit on a vegetarian diet; they were healed when she abstained. So, instead of fruit, in his book, he promised practitioners salvation through two foods alone: peanut oil and cornmeal.

If Cornelius was the only one preaching these kinds of puritanical, scientifically unfounded claims about health, it might be easier to write him off. But Cornelius wasn't isolated in his thinking—his work originated in a time period characterized by changing attitudes about the relationship between health and food. In the late 1800s, refrigerated transport options meant that the price of meat dropped and people from all classes could afford to purchase it, as well as store it in their kitchens at home. As urbanization and industrialization increased, so did fears about the spread of diseases. In the early 1900s, World War I heightened these anxieties even further, as soldiers returned with both physical and mental health issues that medical professionals scrambled to find answers to, through methods that quickly became controversial (like vivisection). While medical advances were broadening resources of care for people experiencing different maladies—including a cure for syphilis, the invention of splints, and acknowledgment of the effect of talk-therapy on mental health—there were still plenty of disorders and illnesses, as well as classes of people who did not have easy access to medicine they fully trusted. As a result, from Britain to South Africa, Australia to the United States, people seeking cures from an assortment of ailments and ills began trying to purify their bodies, and a movement toward a type of vegetarianism steeped in religious morality began.

* * *

In 1887, a woman named Pattie E. Beard (who also went by Annie Patterson) began experiencing a pain that was unrelenting. Her symptoms meant that she was unable to complete her household duties, read for more than ten minutes, or walk. She took a bath chair—a plush, padded version of a contemporary wheelchair—everywhere, and was confronted daily by newspaper ads insisting that she might be healed by products like HUGHES'S BLOOD PILLS! (fixes everything from dyspepsia to nervousness!) and GEORGE'S PILE AND GRAVEL PILLS (as one patient testified, "They saved me from the jaws of death"). Pattie ignored the ads and instead sought care where she thought she would be most likely to receive it: from an eminent physician. Her husband, Sidney Beard, a stockbroker, had hypnotized Pattie during their courtship, both literally and in a romantic sense. He supported her financially as she sought the finest care, but one doctor turned to two, and then to a series of medical men who performed operations on her, prescribed her medication, and left her experiencing the same pain she had been in before. After seven long years of searching for a cure, Pattie fell under a different kind of spell. She and Sidney attended a lecture presented by the Vegetarian Society in Exeter, in which the speaker told the crowd that it was beneficial to live without "flesh-food." From that night on, haunted by the suffering of animals, the couple decided that never again would their "lips be stained with the flesh and blood of our fellow creatures."

At first, their decision was personal. On their new diet, they both felt better. In a column titled "Good News for the Afflicted," Pattie wrote that she sold her bath chair after six months on the diet and took up bicycling instead. As time went on, neither Sidney nor Pattie required medical attention or spent a single day sick in bed. The couple grew enamored with the fleshless, bloodless diet that they believed had cured them of all ills, and they began pressing their newfound way of life on loved ones. When family and friends dined at their house and finished their bowls of soup, they found "Blood and Fire" stamped at the bottom. This served both as a call to Sidney's extra-curricular evangelical work with the Salvation Army and as a marker of his tremendous fervor for his beliefs. He had also decorated his bathrooms and bedrooms with sheets, bath towels, and bathmats inscribed with the Salvation Army's motto. His fanaticism for religion began to meld with his passion for abstaining from meat. His proselytizing soon extended far beyond the walls of his own home in Ilfracombe, a seaside town in England.

At a hotel built atop the Torrs cliffs where he resided, Sidney took visits from leaders in the vegetarian movement, like J. I. Pengelly and Josiah Oldfield. In *The Beacon*, they strategized about how to best spread the good news, and recalled a vegetarian organization founded in 1882 that had lapsed due to a lack in funding. Backed by Sidney's financial power from his years spent stockbroking, The Order of the Golden Age, a vegetarian organization rooted in Christianity, was re-instated in 1895, and the first issue of *The Herald of the Golden Age*, the monthly newsletter of the Order, was published in 1896. Both the organization and newsletter were heavily influenced by cultural context, as well as Christian religion, so the information about vegetarianism was often delivered in a sermonic tone.

As an example, in *The Herald of the Golden Age*, appetite is often intertwined with morality and religion. While rhetorically effective, this connection was nothing new. Rather, in the Christian tradition, linking godliness (or a perceived lack thereof) and consumption harkens all the way back to the first book in the Bible, where Eve succumbs to temptation and eats the forbidden fruit. As religious scholar Michelle

Mary Lelwica writes, "Eve's lack of restraint . . . revealed females' susceptibility to bodily cravings." Saint Augustine of Hippo, using Eve and others as examples, warned Christians not to fall prey to the desires of their flesh, and in Medieval times, Christian ascetics believed that they could be closer to God if they denied themselves any corporeal cravings for food, sex, or even community with others. By emptying their physical bodies, they could make room for the Lord. Hundreds of years later, The Order of the Golden Age took up the principle of abstaining from pleasurable consumption as a means of proving faithfulness—as well as serving as a marker of class—haunting English citizens enough to shape their dietary habits and expectations of appearance in the eighteenth and nineteenth centuries.

Another factor to consider in the Order's mission was its interplay with developing aesthetics of desirability. In 1684, French physician François Bernier published "New Division of the Earth by the Different Species or Races of Man that Inhabit It," which is largely considered the first racial classification system. In his text, as Sabrina Strings explains in *Fearing the Black Body*, Bernier attempted to distinguish Europeans from non-Europeans based on physical qualities, and not without racial bias; Bernier clearly marks so-called "European features" as being superior to any other. Because of his classification system and the numerous responses published by other white European men in the years that followed, Strings writes, "The racialized female body became legible, a form of 'text' from which racial superiority and inferiority were read." While once white women had been celebrated for their full figures (Albrecht Dürer's 1528 renderings of a "normal" woman feature curves and a plump posterior), from 1680-1815, "It was becoming part of the general zeitgeist that fatness was related to blackness. Thus, it was treated as evidence of barbarism, of a nonwhite affectation." Religious leaders, physicians, and philosophers alike chimed in with their thoughts on what "well-mannered women and men should eat," and much of their advice suggested that forgoing food and showing self-restraint (both through appetite and through thinness) was most becoming.

Influenced by a combination of Christian asceticism, the insidious strain of racist depictions of African women that had flooded English "scientific" literature at the time, and the physical effects of English citizens having access to more sugar and alcohol than ever before, new forms of fad dieting were born. While not all practitioners at the time would readily cite any moral, religious, or racist influences, the diets and their urgings were certainly shaped by such cultural forces. One example of this is Dr. George Cheyne, who originally thought he would end up as a man of the Church before switching career paths to medicine. After studying with Scottish physician Sir Archibald Pitcairn, he applied and was accepted as a Fellow of the Royal Society in 1702. There, Cheyne threw himself into his studies—and into a life of partying. His friends in school were a group of "bottle-companions, the younger gentry, and free-livers," and because of his time spent sedentary, studying, soon his weight swelled. A mirthful, kind, and humorous man by all written accounts, Cheyne, after earning his medical title, often met with patients in coffeehouses and split his time "betwixt his patients and the punchbowl." His lifestyle caught up to him. He "grew excessively fat, short-breath'd, lethargic and listless" and suffered from "numerous illnesses, including autumnal intermittent fever, vertiginous paroxysm, vertigo, constant violent headaches, giddiness, lowness, anxiety, and terror." Rather than offer Cheyne aid, his friends "dropt off like autumnal leaves" and continued partying without him.

Alone and unable to cure his own ailing body despite his medical training, Cheyne took a step back from his practice and moved by himself to the country. There, he tried purging both body and soul. He took mercury to induce vomiting and spent a lot of time contemplating how he had been living. He recognized that he had been chasing "sensual Pleasures" and "mere Jollity" rather than following God's will for his life. It was here, at his lowest spiritually and physically, that a surprising cure was delivered to him by an anonymous doctor: a milk diet. For some time, Cheyne exclusively drank milk and ate fruit and vegetables. In his own words, he became "lank, fleet, and nimble," and returned to his practice, where he not only offered patients treatments for their ailments but also spread the gospel of milk. Cheyne's influence seems to have been strong enough to influence, as Strings writes, "a wide swath of haute English women." One of these women, Lady Mary Wortley Montagu, lost weight by drinking "half a pint of warm asses' milk" in the morning and "another dose of asses' milk" at night.

While the milk diet ended up not working out long term for Cheyne—he started drinking two or three pints of wine a day, ate large dinners, and his weight climbed to 448 pounds—the experiment *did* shape the way he viewed food. Rather than continuing to swing from one extreme diet to another, Cheyne allowed himself to enjoy "milk, tea, coffee, bread, butter, mild cheese, fruits, nuts and tender 'roots', including potatoes, turnips, and carrots." He no longer consumed wine or liquor, but sometimes allowed himself "a glass of soft small cider." In comparison to his punchbowl days, he felt like a new man. He wanted others to feel well, too, so he published *An Essay of Health and Long Life*, which outlined his recommendations: moderate exercise, eight ounces of meat and twelve ounces of vegetable for an ordinary man who doesn't do much manual labor, and no overuse of alcohol—though he makes clear he is not against "enlivening conversation, promoting friendship, comforting the sorrowful heart, and raising the drooping spirits by the cheerful cup." He emphasized a vegetable-forward menu but left room for practitioners to eat meat in moderation. For someone writing in 1724, Cheyne's treatise, which emphasizes prevention rather than miracle cures, is not bad—or at least better than the milk diet.

Cheyne's writings left a meaningful impact on other thinkers who followed, and the idea of vegetarianism took root in Great Britain in the early 1800s. Eager to share the benefits, both in terms of improving their health and relieving their consciences, vegetarians at the time published essays, articles, and books about their dietary choices. Sir Richard Phillips, in 1811, made a list of sixteen reasons to take up a vegetarian diet, which includes abstaining from refining "the most cruel practices of the most savage animals [of other species]" or "*bleeding, skinning, roasting, and boiling animals alive, and torturing them without reservation or remorse*, if they thereby add to the variety or the delicacy of their carnivorous gluttony" (italic emphasis courtesy of Sir Phillips). Others, like John Frank Newton, emphasized positive personal health benefits. "Having for many years been a habitual invalid," Newton writes, "and having at length found that relief from regimen which I had long and vainly hoped for from drugs . . . I [now] enjoy an existence which many might envy who consider themselves to be in full possession of the blessings of health."

One man in particular, who was influenced both by "the medical arguments of Dr. Cheyne and the humanitarian sentiments of St. Pierre," was Reverend William Cowherd, who founded the Bible Christian Church. Ironically, considering his name, Cowherd made people sign an agreement promising to abstain from eating animals to be considered members of his parish. Though Cowherd passed in 1816, his Cowherdites, as they called themselves, drove forward. In 1817, a group of two ministers, twenty adults, and nineteen children left England on a ship and endured an eleven-week journey to Philadelphia. While they traveled there to spread the gospel of abstinence from meat and alcohol in the United States, many of them lost sight of their goal once they arrived. Impoverished, earning "their daily bread by the sweat of their brows," and isolated from one another in a foreign country, they gave up their vegetarianism and simply tried to survive. But there was one small flock of Cowherdites who stuck to their principles: Reverend James Clark, who purchased land in Lycoming County, Pennsylvania, and Reverend William Metcalfe, who stayed committed to his diet in spite of yellow fever, poverty, and offers from friends to help him if he would eat meat once more. Metcalfe published "The Duty of Abstinence from all Intoxicating Drinks" and "Abstinence from the Flesh of Animals," which he insists were the first motion toward temperance in the United States, and his work paved the way for others to publish vegetarian cookbooks and texts.

In England, where many Cowherdites had remained, one of Cowherd's former pupils, Joseph Brotherton, met with five other men between the ages of fifty-seven and eighty, all of whom "looked truly patriarchal, healthy, strong, and full of intelligence and love." But their looks weren't all that united them; each man had been vegetarian anywhere from thirty-three to thirty-eight years, and they had come together to encourage everyone in the world to become vegetarian, to work toward "true civilization, to universal brotherhood, and to the increase of human happiness generally." On the morning of September 30, 1847, they gathered in Northwood Villa, a towering, castle-like structure that doubled as a hydropathy institution in the seaside town of Ramsgate. These six men knew that God had given to man "every herb bearing seed" ("Hear, hear"), that eating meat was a sign of a "depraved appetite" ("Hear, hear, and cheers"), and that eating vegetables rather than meat had made them "better and stronger" than they had ever been before" ("Hear"). Without irony, these men testified that "the world was [their] country, and to do good [their] religion" ("Hear, hear, and cheers").

The men believed it was their duty to spread the word, and so— through publications, books, and a lecture series—they converted others to a flesh-free diet. Through one of the many lectures presented by the society, Pattie and Sidney Beard would be lured in by the promise of health.

*   *   *

In an excerpt from *Metamorphoses*, featured in *Fruits and Farinacea: The Proper Food of Man*, by Vegetarian Society member John Smith, Ovid writes:

Not so the golden age, who fed on fruit,
Nor durst with bloody meals their mouths pollute.
Then birds in airy space might safely move,
And tim'rous hares on heaths securely rove:
Nor needed fish the guileful hooks to fear,
For all was peaceful; and that peace sincere.

Ovid's emphasis on peacefulness in regard to abstaining from meat-eating is a worthy vision, but one that did not come to fruition, at least not in nineteenth century Great Britain. Instead, vegetarians were plagued with infighting. The Vegetarian Society split into two factions in 1888: the London Vegetarian Society, which was more stringent, and the Manchester Vegetarian Society, in which President Francis William Newman allowed members to occasionally eat fish. For a new vegetarian group to enter the scene successfully and gain members, it needed to up the ante.

When The Order of the Golden Age was founded in 1895, it did just that. Rather than refer to themselves as "vegetarians" like the other groups, they coined the term "fruitarian." While contemporarily the word "fruitarian" usually refers to someone who lives only on raw fruit (with some possible exceptions for greens or nuts), the word within the context of the Order allowed followers to eat vegetables, fruits, cereals, cooked food, and even dairy and eggs. At the time, by using fruitarian as a descriptor, the Order hoped to distinguish their diet from the "faddism" of vegetarianism, as they considered their "sphere of work" to be "amongst a different class of people." In some ways, it can be said that their rebranding of vegetarianism was successful, at least in softening the public's opinion. In a 1914 issue of the *Herald*, Sidney Beard remarked, "When the Order of the Golden Age was founded in 1895 vegetarianism was ridiculed in almost every newspaper in this country, and regarded as a mild form of insanity in almost every home. Now almost every public journal is sympathetic, and many are co-operating with us." While of course Beard's comments about his own organization should be taken with a grain of salt, the 1929 edition of the *Encyclopedia Britannica* confirms the influence of the Order, stating, "Since about 1901, the Order of the Golden Age has come to the front" of vegetarian societies.

This is where things get thorny. Convinced of the moral sanctity of their fruitarianism, the leaders of The Order of the Golden Age not only continued proselytizing in England, but also set up international headquarters in Natal, South Africa. There, in a report that reeks of colonialism, the "Pioneers of the Order of the Golden Age" gave "lectures to natives" and offered "a Christmas appeal concerning humane diet." Echoing the racist travelogues and race classification systems of the time, there are also articles in the *Herald* that celebrate the conversion of "mostly natives who had been converted from carnivorism," though "these native reformers 'were admittedly the best specimens of their race.'"

Rather than just offering relief to the populace from "joints and tissues . . . choked by waste and uric acid," or "the demon Gout and his malign kindred" through a diet alternative to the meat-heavy norm in England at the time, the Order stressed that they were offering people salvation from moral failings as well—all through food. They believed that eating meat was "the cause of a large proportion of the Pain, Disease, Suffering, and Depravity with which our race is cursed." While I'm sure that a vegetarian diet does work in some people's lifestyles and help them feel better and happier, articles in the *Herald* in no way take into account cultural practices, class, disability, or access to food that might influence diet. The rhetoric of the Order began to lean toward individual responsibility for wellness. In an article titled "Hygienic Christianity," Sidney Beard writes that "real followers" of Christ should feel obligated to "relieve human suffering," and that it was each person's responsibility to purify themselves through food in order to prevent disease as well as cure it.

The problem with purity is that there is never an end to it, rarely a way to reasonably quantify how pure something is, and at worst, it is a word loaded with racist, classist, sexist moral ideals. The *Herald's* proclamation that "the great scientific fact that purity of food tends to promote purity of Character," or Dr. J. Kellogg's insistence that "for the making of pure blood, the first essential is pure food," sets up a false promise of wellness that practitioners then spent days, weeks, months, or—in the case of Essie Honiball—their lives chasing. Insisting on purity as a necessity pitted practitioners against their own willpower: If they could not keep up with the fruitarian diet, it was their shortcoming, and any illness, weight gain, or moral fault after that could be attributed to their lack of commitment to the "right" diet and the thin path of salvation offered by Christian leaders. And worse, if they committed entirely to the preaching of a teacher who had no real credentials, they might lose their health—or their life.

CHAPTER 5

I Shall Be Healed

I IMAGINE THAT FOR ESSIE, IN THE WEEKS SHE WAS withholding food from herself, there might have been a satisfying sort of discomfort that gnawed at her throughout the day, an underlying buzz in her body distracting her from emotional layers of hurt. Or maybe I'm just imposing my own theories about self-harm on her story because it's easier than examining my own.

The morning after my run on the train tracks, I felt angry when I woke up. Ahead of me was another day with too many hours in which I might succumb to symptoms, run into a former teammate, or simply ache from the loss that thrummed through me like a current: no more team, no more team, no more team. I was electric with a desire for pain. I wanted to punish myself for the ways my body had failed me. That night, my roommate Eliza walked into my room and offered me tenderness. She sat with me while I confessed that I had run away the night before, coaxed me into making a counseling appointment, and left a note beneath my door before the following dawn: *Jacqueline, if you are reading this before the sun has come up, turn around and get back into bed.*

You matter to me. In fact, you matter to a lot of people. And you're awesome.
And things will get better. Pinky swear.

Eliza's kindness kept me alive, but I wasn't ready at the time to fully heal, or even to reckon meaningfully with my past. Instead, I found other ways of moderating my feelings. I continued cutting myself and lied to my counselor until they relieved me from making any future appointments. When I heard the word *whale* haunting me when I looked in the mirror, I adopted my former teammate's disgust as my own: I took half of a double-layer chocolate cake that Eliza and I had baked to a parking lot and ate until my stomach was distended. I ate a full jar of peanut butter behind the locked door of my room, telling myself that the habit was better than cutting. I ate and ate and ate, not for pleasure or nourishment, but to numb myself. I ate until the potential for joy became nothing but a heavy ache.

I continued sneaking away, too, though this time in broad daylight. While at the start of the semester I had made Eliza maps of where my runs would take me and confided in her that I was scared one day I might become episodic during my daily miles, I began running without telling anyone where I was going or how long I'd be gone. One day, I pressed the "Start" button on my watch, lifted my right foot from the ground, then left, then right, left, right, the comforting music of rubber soles against concrete carrying me away from the apartment, past the track complex, across a big intersection, and out onto the farmland roads. We had run there once as a team, but girls from the flat Midwest complained that the run was too hilly, so we never ran it again. Without the team around me to buffer my body from oncoming traffic, and without a captain to tell me where to go, the farmlands seemed uncharted, a place I could make my mark. Mile one was a long straight stretch of road where an old shed crumbled into itself like rotten fruit, a concrete wall showed its age in a jagged crack, and a deer carcass hung bloody from a large oak tree. Mile two was a house with wood siding peeling away from the frame, roosters crowing in the late afternoon, fruitless vines of muscadine grapes. A herd of sienna-colored cows pressed their wet noses against the fence when I ran past, their dark eyes following me.

Just down the hill from the cows was the three-mile mark. I slowed in the middle of the lane and hit the "Stop" button on my wrist. The sun warmed my shoulders, and there was no one around. Not even the whine of a faraway car penetrated the silence. I walked slowly across the street toward a house. Bushes grew wild at the front, clambering up to the second-story window panes. Each brick of the grey two-story home was stamped with a star, all of them at a slightly different angle. There was no car in front, no sign of anyone living there, so I walked up to the side of the house, my heart pounding in my chest. I reached out and grazed the rough surface of one of the bricks with my fingertips. To my left was a shed made from corrugated aluminum that stood as tall as the home, a worn wooden ladder propped against the entryway. There was another low shed behind the home, one with wide enough gaps between the wooden slats that I could decipher the shimmer of a line of colored glass bottles, their blues and greens refracting like ocean water.

A tall tree blocked the sun for a moment and a shadow swooped over me. I whirled from left to right, looking over each shoulder as if someone might be behind me. Maybe the house wasn't abandoned. The blinds were closed in each window, but the blinds of the left back room on the top floor were cracked open, like an angular gap between off-white teeth. My heart pattered and I ran back to the open road, pressed "Start" on my watch, and took a right at the stop sign, away from campus. While my first few runs after quitting the team had felt trivial, this run seemed different. I felt a release. Part of that came from a dark impulse, a taunt, that perhaps I would become episodic on these roads, that I would be hauled into the back of a strange truck or that my body would be flattened like an opossum I'd stopped to examine, innards pointing in the direction she might have been traveling.

But there was a glimmer of something good that came over me, too. I found myself delighted when my legs burned, lungs searing with their work. The run didn't feel trite like my neighborhood jogs; even though I didn't have a clipboard to chart my progress, I felt strength in the way I moved forward.

I took note of the scenery as I ran. A pond—surface so still it begged to be broken—was mile five. Mile six was marked by a red-roofed cabin with a yard of garden gnomes lined up like a choir. Mile seven was two yowling dogs. Eight was the rolling back fields of a prison farm, enclosed by barbed wire and electricity. Nine was the spindly limbs of apple trees. Ten was dirt piles of an unfinished job, and a dock no one jumped from. Near the end of mile ten, I reached a T-intersection. Cars whizzed by and gravel sprayed from the back of a truck. Late autumn humidity roiled from the pavement.

I turned back the way I had come and jogged slowly along the side of the road. My quads ached with the task of lifting, and my calves throbbed. When I looked down, my legs looked swollen, the skin tight and warm to the touch. I liked the idea that I was pushing myself to my limits. The last mile of the run was largely uphill, and I felt myself straining against the incline. My legs were dull with fatigue. I couldn't think of anything but step-step-step again now step-step-step. My armpits rubbed raw against my cotton T-shirt. Sunlight glistened orange between boughs ahead, and I urged myself onward, telling myself there would be food at home. Water. Shower. Sleep. I muscled through the last half mile and bent over outside of the apartment. Without meaning to, I smiled. My limbs were wracked with an immense ache, but I felt pleasure in the fact that I had controlled my own debilitation. No episode had snatched away my ability to stand, no man had carried me to safety, no doctor had measured the beat of my heart. I had reclaimed part of myself, it seemed.

When I unlocked the door, my roommates asked, "*Where have you been? Are you okay?*" I answered vaguely that I had been out in the farmlands. I smiled at Eliza, who had a worried look on her face. I glugged water and brought a glass to the bathroom, feeling simultaneous manic excitement and physical exhaustion as I turned the knob of the shower, steam slowly ascending from the tub. My legs trembled as I stepped in. I stood for a moment. Breathed in the steam. Let the water saturate my hair. Caressed my skin gently for the first time in a long time while I washed: fingertips dabbing soap near my wrists, stroking away rough clusters of salt from my jawline.

*   *   *

During my freshman-year semester when I first began having episodes, one of my nonsensical refrains was "Aurora." *Aurora, Aurora, Auror-ror-ror-a, Aurora.* The name of a princess who, at sixteen, pricks her finger and falls into such a deep sleep that it's almost as if she doesn't belong to her body anymore. The period before Prince Phillip kisses her is lost. But, of course, Aurora wakes up—or is awoken by a nonconsensual kiss—from her slumber. She and the prince waltz off to a ball. She lives happily ever after; no trauma from the forgotten days of her life and no lasting effects—at least none we are made aware of—from a stranger kissing her.

My sleep was not so easy. No matter how many miles I ran in a day—often twenty down the farmland roads—or how safe I felt in my apartment watching TV with Eliza, nights brought back terrors from some half-submerged place. Shortly after drifting off, I would feel someone's lips pressing against mine. The lips were clammy and firm, real enough that I would thrash back and forth as if to fight someone off me, before realizing I was alone. I would then get up, check the lock on my door and the narrow space below my bed. Even when all was secure, I would still be so shaken—by the dream, by the memory, by the feeling that was both a memory and a nightmare—that I would stay awake, crying and tense, too alarmed to fall back into any sort of comfortable sleep.

Unable to quell my urges to self-harm, I alternated between long runs through the farmlands, overeating, and cutting myself most of my sophomore fall semester. I wore sweatshirts to class even in warm weather to cover my arms and stayed silent in the back row of classes— still terrified, in spite of the medication, that I would lose my voice to illness. I sweated and shifted through every lecture, wanting to be on the road or in my room, losing myself to whatever particular pain might soothe me that day. The depression felt like a bottomless chasm, one that left me feeling powerless as I stood at the edge. Mid-semester, my mom flew from Oklahoma to North Carolina to visit me, and the balancing act of our calls unraveled. Over the phone line, I could pretend to be okay, but not when she saw me. Wanting more answers than the half-truths I had given, my mom accompanied me to the neurologist. He was in one of his quiet moods that day, no caroling of symptoms, no melodic *how are you.* He asked if there was anything new.

"Not much," I said. I looked down at my palms. "The medication makes me feel cloudy, I think, but I feel okay in regard to symptoms."

"You shouldn't be feeling cloudy on the medication," he said. "Are you sure that you're not just tired?"

Ashamed that I again felt what I shouldn't, I nodded. "You're right," I said. "I'm sure starting school again is just getting to me."

"Tell him about the . . ." my mom hesitated. "Tell him about the depression."

"Depression?" the doctor stopped fumbling for his instruments.

"It's nothing," I said. "I've been . . . well, I've been, uh, cutting myself."

"Cutting?"

"Yes, cutting. I feel depressed and I cut myself," I explained. "I am seeing a counselor, and everything is fine."

"Could the medication be causing her depression?" my mom asked. Her ballpoint pen was poised above a yellow legal pad. The doctor stroked his scruff.

"Hmm," he mused. "I don't think so."

My mom nodded. The doctor tapped on each of my knees with a metal hammer, asked me to walk across the room, and asked me to speak. I performed normally in each of the tests. His conjecture based on my physical appearance seemed reminiscent of the athletic trainer's refrain of *she's okay, she's okay* each time my blood pressure and heart rate came back in normal ranges. If I looked okay, if I achieved normal results on tests when asked, then I was fine. Nothing to diagnose.

During the appointment, even though my mom raised the question about my medication, Keppra, influencing my mood, the doctor dismissed her concern. In his notes, however, he wrote "Depression onset after starting Keppra 500 mg twice a day. Must conclude mood effects may be due to Keppra. However, this has helped resolve her seizure type activity." Rather than disclosing this information and asking whether or not I wanted to wean off of Keppra or try an alternate seizure medication, the doctor suggested that I continue taking the same dose and "Consider for Antidepressant trial" as well. He suggested a psychiatrist.

In the office, seated on the crinkly paper of the patient table, I disregarded my intuition. Maybe I was making it all up. Maybe I was just emotional. Maybe I had broken under the pressure of being a Division I Athlete. I made excuses for my condition, all of them my fault. I wonder now how many months of darkness I might have been spared had my mom and I pushed harder in that appointment to establish a connection between the medication and my intense depression. Though I know that my low state was due in part to me quitting the team and my unresolved feelings about what had happened to me on my mattress on the floor, I have never in my life felt as wildly out of control as I did while on Keppra. When put on the same medication six years later, while in my PhD program, I would again experience suicidal thoughts and feel the urge to self-harm. I knew enough the second time to alert my doctor, who listened to me rather than dismissing my emotional state as being something less real than my physical one.

But that day, the doctor assured me that the medication was sup-
pressing any abnormalities. He told me to continue with my dosage,
and sent my mom and me on our way, no need for a follow-up for
months. My mom left days later. When I went to see the psychiatrist
that the neurologist had recommended, he prescribed me an antidepressant, and I took it. Like some backwards version of Aurora, I started
sleeping thirteen or fourteen hours a night. I was not running anymore
and not cutting anymore and not feeling anything anymore. It was
comforting and terrible all at once. Months passed. Outside my bedroom window, pink flowers bloomed. There was no prince coming to
wake me.

*   *   *

I had only experienced one breakthrough episode since starting the
seizure medication nearly a year before, so at my final neurology
appointment of the semester, I requested that the doctor take me off both
the seizure medication and the antidepressants. As counterproductive
as it might seem on the surface, I was operating under the logic that
the neurologist himself had offered when he first met me: At eighteen,
my brain was still malleable enough that he hoped a short stint on
medication could correct the neurons; it was never supposed to be long-
term. He agreed. I stopped taking medication.

At the end of the semester, instead of returning home to live with
my family for the summer, I moved to Columbia, Missouri, where I
had secured an internship at a literary magazine. I moved into a dormitory room below ground. From my room's slim window, only a mulch
bed was visible. My mom helped me unpack the few belongings I'd
brought with me. Before leaving, she looked me in the eye. "You'll
call if you need us, right?" she asked. "We're trusting you." I nodded.
Secretly, I was delirious at the idea of freedom. No one in the whole city
knew anything about me. No Eliza to make sure I came home, no one

who could recognize me if I had an episode, no medication smothering my symptoms. I held a perverse belief that I needed to be alone to truly know I had healed.

In theory, being by myself seemed exciting—but after my mom left, my dorm room felt dismal: concrete floors painted gray, a stained mattress covered by my sheets, the rattle of the air conditioner kicking on every once in a while. Each day, bound only by a few hours of waitressing and infrequent magazine meetings, I passed time with exercise. I spent hours watching TV on the screen of an elliptical machine in the gym. On runs outside, I spooked at the sound of another's footsteps. I woke up earlier than most students on campus so I could sit alone at breakfast and eat as little as possible. I kept a calorie counter in an Excel sheet and kept myself going on Fiber One bars and cucumbers from the cafeteria. I willed my body into oblivion.

I walked everywhere that summer: to the Thai restaurant where I worked, to the coffee shop, to the magazine's headquarters, to the dining hall. A buzzing sound persisted no matter where I went. The skies grew black with the bulbous bodies of cicadas. Trees lit up in great thrums of activity, bushes rustled.

Thousands of cicada shells were frozen against the bark of campus trees, all forever clambering toward the top branches. The skeletons were flawless casts of the cicadas that had left them, each leg clinging to the tree exactly as the cicada had positioned it, each rounded outline of an eye still visible on the empty shell. Each evening, I watched the cicadas wriggle away from themselves. They seemed to understand what it's like to leave a part of yourself behind, to see the shape of your own empty body, your exoskeleton a home you can never fit back into or fill up again.

It might have been because I was so far from campus, so distant from the team and a couple years away from my first collapse, but I became obsessed with the insects. The whole town did: A local ice cream shop sold out of cicada ice cream before the flavor was shut down by the health department; campus maintenance swept thousands of bodies from the sidewalks; I read in the local paper that the insects were producing a sound louder than a rock concert or a jet engine. I batted the creatures away when they bumbled toward my head but rejoiced in their persistent screams. I imagined them yelling, *We're alive! There is sunlight!* In contrast, I stayed in my basement dorm room, called my parents each day to tell them I was fine, and worked the elliptical until my legs were numb. I was healthy, at least physically, but felt haunted by my body's own history.

In the months I lived alone, I started wriggling free from the griefs that had calcified around me. While I still had a long road of healing ahead in terms of my relationship to my body, I began to see the beauty in shedding some hard external layer to reveal tenderness. After a year spent hiding in my apartment, staying silent in class, and sleeping days away, I began to imagine what it might look like to let myself want something again: relationships with new friends; letting people hear my voice, even if I feared the sounds that might someday again emerge; and running on my own terms. I enrolled in writing classes at my university. I signed up for a marathon. I watched as the cicadas let their soft selves emerge from their shells into the light. They twirled in the face of uncertainty and sang.

CHAPTER 6

Guinea Pigs, Gurus, and People in Pain

AFTER ABOUT A MONTH ON THE FRUIT DIET, ESSIE GREW A little bit stronger. She still experienced envy when she walked past cafes and saw people eating her old favorite foods, but she was heartened by how the fruit experiment made her feel. A skin rash that had swept over her body suddenly disappeared. Her sinus pains vanished. Cornelius informed her that her "bloodstream had been purged of the substances (or 'misplaced material' . . .) that had polluted it and caused [her] illness." Unlike other people, who ate toxins and died in sin, Essie was ridding herself of "poisons," "impurities," "mucus," and "contamination." Rather than view Essie's growing healthfulness as relief, or as an opportunity to slowly introduce new foods back into her diet, Cornelius most likely echoed advice he had communicated through his book, *The Bible of Nature*, years before. "'NO COMPROMISE' if you wish to succeed . . . Say

'NO COMPROMISE' to yourselves the last thing every night, and the first thing every morning. And mean it when you say it."

And what shouldn't people compromise on, according to Cornelius? No alcohol, opium, whisky, tea, or coffee. No stimulating foods, for they cause "sexual excesses and abuses." No frying food, for it destroys food value. No high-protein food, as it has been known to cause "hyper-sexuality" in monkeys, at least the ones he visited once in a zoo. High-protein foods are as sinful as "bashing in your wife's head or her nagging at you in a state of nervous and mental derangement." No insulin for diabetics, as it just poisons you further. No prayer can make you purer; some passages in the Bible "are so filthy I doubt whether even a hardened prostitute would care to read it to her associates." And certainly, if you are ill, do *not*, under any circumstance, visit a doctor. According to Dr. J. M. Good, as cited in Cornelius's book, "Medicine has destroyed more lives than war, pestilence, and famine combined." And according to Dr. A. M. Rose, "The medical system is a colossal deception that has filled the world with incurable invalids, for which mines have been emptied of cankering minerals, the intestines of animals taxed for their filth, the poison-bags of reptiles drained of their venom, the blood of cats and dogs extracted, and all these with other abominations have been thrust down the throat of gullible human beings." Doctors are silly little pet Satans, Cornelius says, who just desire money and professional kudos. There's no actual healing to be found in the field of medicine.

While some of these commandments are stamped with Cornelius's signature bombastic style, a lot of these ideas really weren't all that original, especially considering the time period. Some of them can be traced back to the rhetoric found within publications like *The Herald of the Golden Age*, in which symptoms of illness were seen as signs of sin, or a lapse in good dietary or religious judgment. But the movement toward vegetarianism doesn't necessarily explain Cornelius's specific obsession with peanut oil and cornmeal during his early years in Australia or how—and why—after his years on the peanut oil circuit, he shifted away from it. Where did he get the idea that fruit might help Essie heal? The answer might come from a field of alternative medical healers that Cornelius once dismissed as "food cranks" and "quacks": naturopaths.

*   *   *

In the late nineteenth century, licensed, formally educated doctors began to standardize and professionalize their techniques and treatment plans. A constellation of populations—Germanic practitioners; women; individuals like Pattie Beard, who were wracked by mysterious illnesses; spiritual healers; and people like Cornelius, who proclaimed themselves to be "doctors" despite having no training—sought alternatives to modern medical practices. Alternative healers offered treatments like sun cures, fasting, hypnotism, herbalism, and hydrotherapy. Though sometimes the nature of their practices differed, their work was united by an underlying belief that each of our bodies has the power to heal itself, if only we don't interfere with "nature."

Benedict Lust, whose body was afflicted by illness, is someone who put his faith in alternative methods of healing. Born in Michelbach, Germany, in 1872, Lust traveled to the United States when he was twenty. He wasn't just sightseeing; he was seeking a cure for tuberculosis, which he claimed was caused by half a dozen vaccines that had been administered to him in his youth. In the US, Lust claimed he appeared so weak that doctors preemptively filled out a death certificate upon seeing him. (No evidence of this death certificate has been located.) Wasting away, devastated by the doctors who had disappointed him after such a long journey, Lust returned to Germany. There, he abandoned modern medicine for a stay with Father Sebastian Kneipp. Kneipp, who preached moderate exercise, simple foods that weren't too spicy, herbs, and taking early walks barefoot in the morning dew, was well known for his alternative approach to healing. He administered a series of "cold water" treatments to Lust, who recovered from his tuberculosis after eight months.

Kneipp died the year after, but his philosophy toward the body lived on through Lust, who returned to the United States in 1894 raring to share new ways of natural healing. Worried that the public would be scared off by the sight of patients wandering Central Park barefoot at dawn, Lust eliminated some of Kneipp's cures and added his own. He dispensed dietetic advice, gave chiropractic adjustments and massages, and used water, homeopathy, and light to treat patients. While there were other practitioners like Lust who used an eclectic set of therapies, it took a while for them to organize and find a name. Legend has it that after working with hygienic healer Dr. Sophie Scheel at the Homeopathic College in New York City, Lust burst into a colleague's office and announced, "We now have a name for our work!"

Women, vegetarians, religious devotees, spiritual and mental healers, and anti-vaccinationists who felt like outsiders gathered beneath the proverbial banner of the newly minted naturopathy. They began to share information, both informally and publicly, to circumvent the medical systems in place. For populations who had been dismissed or ignored by trained doctors, these methods allowed them to feel a modicum of control over their healing and to believe in the inherent goodness of their bodies. Much like the moralistic, religious overtones that seep into the pages of The Order of the Golden Age's newsletter, naturopathy also placed blame on individuals if they fell ill or if symptoms recurred. Symptoms were a sign that patients had not been "pure" enough or that they had allowed the evils of the world to infiltrate their bodies. Christian-based vegetarians and naturopathic practitioners shared such similar values, both health-wise and morality-wise, that the two fields began to intertwine in ways both productive and problematic.

Beneficially—at least for vegetarians and naturopathic practitioners at the time—as naturopathy grew as a field, The Order of the Golden

Age extended support in the form of advertisements and articles featuring new "natural" methodologies, treatments, and testimonials in their newsletter. Someone picking up an issue of *The Herald of the Golden Age* in 1897 to learn more about vegetarianism would have also encountered terminology related to early forms of naturopathy, like "Hygienic and Natural Law," which encouraged them to partake in only "pure food, pure water, and pure air." They would have seen advertisements for places like the Clevedon Hydropathic Establishment, where they might stay in a ventilated, mild environment full of winter sunshine to cure "Insomnia, Dyspepsia, Gout, Rheumatism, and Pulmonary Affections." While surely a bit of sunshine and fresh air might have provided relief for some patients, these articles and advertisements feature no disclaimer from medical professionals about potential negative side effects, and no scientific evidence to back up their cures. And that was the point. In fact, news briefings in the *Herald* went further, imbuing scientific studies with a negative moral connotation. In a criticism of experimentation on animals that a professor was conducting in the hopes of finding a cure for yellow fever, an English physician, Dr. Berdoe, is quoted, with emphasis his own, as saying, *"Deliberate murder* can be committed in a laboratory for scientific purposes." In another briefing, a man named Dr. Clifford is summarized saying, again with his own emphasis, that *"unhealthy* people physically, tend to become an *immoral* people." Whoever read the *Herald* looking for nutrition advice might have found it but would have also seen public health policy and science skewed as immoral, sinful pursuits rather than as scientifically-based efforts—conducted by highly trained individuals—to make advances in medicine that might save large swaths of people.

While naturopaths themselves might have celebrated a space where they could make claims about health that supported their worldview, their rejection of evidence-based healing methods and medical systems meant that they were very reluctant to create any regulatory body for their own field. This made an easy entry for charlatans to slip in and swindle patients, as well as get off scot-free for their transgressions. (As when Cornelius "Robert" Valkenberg de Villiers Dreyer served just six months for his role in the death of a man and was back on stage preaching medical advice for hundreds of people just months later.) To separate themselves from the growing crowd of practitioners and to sell both themselves and their merchandise (supplements, stays in sanitariums, publications, books, etc.), naturopathic healers began advertising diets that became more and more extreme.

*   *   *

This extremism is where fruit comes in. While The Order of the Golden Age had once touted a moderate "fruitarian" diet of cereals, nuts, vegetables, and fruits as being the healthiest, whispers of the kind of diet we associate with fruitarianism now, where followers eat raw fruit and only fruit, started to proliferate. More than a permanent lifestyle, the idea of fruitarianism started out as a fad diet masquerading as medical treatment. For example, Benedict Lust used fruit as a form of healing at his health resorts. A jingle for one of these resorts, located just outside New York City, lays bare some of his healing methodologies:

> Mister Lust can make you well,
> if you will let him lay
> The plans for what you eat and
> wear, and his commands obey.
> He's got an Eden out of town,
> where you will get no meat,
> And walk 'mid trees as Adam
> did, in birthday suit complete;
> . . . Roast beef, cigars, and lager-beer
> you'll never want again,

When you've been healed at
[Yungborn], by fruit, fresh air and rain.
It's very cheap as well as good—
this wondrous Nature Cure,
And if you take it home with
you, its blessings will endure;
For all the ills of all mankind,
the cheapest and the best
Is Mister Lust's great Nature
Cure—just put it to the test!

Mister Lust wasn't the only one pairing naturopathic techniques like walking nude outside in fresh air or rain with an all-fruit diet. One of the first mentions of an all-fruit diet appears in the 1897 issue of the *Herald*. Dr. M. L. Holbrook, a prominent American Natural Hygienist, eugenicist, and physician (who believed, among other things, in strength training as a means of lessening people's "morbid craving for unnatural and unreasonable indulgence of the passional nature") wrote about a phenomenon called "the grape cure." What was it supposed to cure? His article doesn't specify, but Holbrook *does* include a litany of rules for how someone should carry out the treatment:

The grapes must be completely ripe.
The grapes must be washed, to rid them of impurities.
The grapes should not be bitten with the teeth but pressed against the roof of the mouth.
The seeds and the skins of the grape should not be swallowed.
The patient must exercise in open air while eating one to two pounds of grapes.
Sometimes, it is okay for a patient to eat a crust of bread between grape servings.

Despite the dearth of information in this particular article, the grape cure was popular enough at the time—at least for alternative-health enthusiasts—for other doctors and facilities to incorporate it into their treatment plans. In 1860, for example, Jean Charles Herpin, a French doctor, published his findings that grape juice "is a kind of vegetable milk, the chemical composition has the greatest analogy with that of woman's milk," and urged people to make sure that this "herbal tea sweetened by nature herself" was a significant part of their diet. In the early 1900s, spurred on by the kind of advice published by Herpin and others, trendy health resorts in Germany, France, and Italy began offering the grape diet to their wealthy clientele. In one photo of Baden-Baden, a luxurious health resort that catered to clientele like Ivan Turgenev and Marlene Dietrich (and still caters to the likes of Victoria Beckham and the Clintons), a waitress stands outfitted in a knee-length black dress, white apron over top. She gives the camera a stern stare and holds a platter of two wine glasses, one filled with lighter grape juice, the other dark. Behind her, two men outfitted in crisp white chef's coats press grapes into juice in small barrels. Before them, lining the table, are bunches and bunches of plump grapes.

Taking the cure even further, in 1927, a woman named Johanna Brandt set sail from her home in South Africa for the United States armed with the knowledge that grapes—and only grapes—could cure any disease, but especially cancer. She departed from South Africa on the Fourth of July. Though the date was coincidental, she imagined that setting forth for the United States on its Independence Day was fortuitous, for she was bringing to the country information that could lead to people's personal liberation from illness. However, her optimism was quickly dashed. Brandt's travels went so poorly that she didn't arrive in New York City until late November. After she arrived, she walked the city, knocked on the doors of doctors, visited preachers, and wrote editors, trying to spread the good news. But no one wanted to listen.

The story she wanted so desperately to tell, as she later would in her book *The Grape Cure*, went something like this: When Brandt turned forty, her mother died from stomach cancer. This wasn't Brandt's first experience with the disease; there had been a lot of cancer deaths in her father's family. But her mother's death was the most impactful. In her grief, Brandt developed gastric trouble, bilious attacks, stomach ulcers, and began to feel a gnawing pain on the left side of her stomach. She began reflecting on her own diet; like many other people she knew who were raised in South Africa in the late 1800s, Brandt had practically been raised on meat, much of it game harvested by family members. That, she decided, was the source of the problem. Years of meat built up in her stomach had begun fermenting and reeking. Though doctors told her that cancer was not hereditary, she knew they were wrong, and she was almost grateful to feel the pain, to know that cancer might be a form of release from the life she was living. She made promises to herself never to get her possible cancer tested by medical professionals, not to go under the knife of a surgeon, never to take an injection. Instead, though she never confirmed what the source of her stomach pain was, she began treating herself for cancer.

She began by fasting. Her remark on this attempt at healing is that it was "disappointing," but that didn't stop her from fasting again and again *and* persuading her friends and family to fast under her supervision. For Brandt, fasting was kind of a gateway to other forms of natural healing. She tried water cures, sunbathing, and deep breathing. Nothing worked. Nine years into her fasting obsession, she was "beyond the starvation point." In 1920, she experienced a bout of vomiting and purging and brought up a "quantity of half-digested blood." Instead of feeling concerned about her skeletal form or finally seeking treatment for what may or may not be cancer, she continued diagnosing herself. The cause of her symptoms was a growth that had originated in her stomach, but had pushed its way through her diaphragm, toward her heart and lungs. She saw it like "a red octopus feeding on impure blood." In this state, weak and consumed by illness, Brandt discovered grapes, which healed her. They didn't just heal her, they healed everyone—from everything. On grapes, Brandt writes, "the senses become abnormally acute; dim eyes brighten; faded hair takes on new gloss; the lifeless, hopeless voice becomes vibrant, magnetic, and the complexion clears."

After three months in New York City, Brandt finally found a sympathetic ear in none other than Benedict Lust, who connected her to Bernarr Macfadden, the editor of the magazine *Physical Culture*. While Brandt might not have delivered the entire United States from "disease and premature death," she did reach a variety of naturopaths, one of whom treated an Englishman, Basil Shackleton, and recommended he read *The Grape Cure*. (In an appendix to his book, Shackleton writes that he eventually got to meet Brandt in person and described her as a "remarkable old lady" who wrote a "little book.") Shackleton wrote about how a "microscopic bug with snout like a corkscrew" had swum up his penis in Africa at a young age, and had lived within him for a while, pockmarking his kidneys from the inside. He began experiencing bouts of pain that radiated from his kidney "through the whole length of the ureter until its reached the testicles." Somehow the bilharzia bug pain transformed to kidney stones (like Brandt, Shackleton seemed to be a fan of self-diagnosis) and Shackleton underwent surgery, after which he bled for three days and was forced into emergency surgery to "staunch the flow of blood and save the life which was fast leaving my young and helpless body." His troubles with health in childhood cast an inauspicious aura over his adulthood. His right kidney was removed by a doctor (upon reflection, Shackleton wishes he would have known about the grape cure back then, as he believes it would have spared him from medical treatment) and his renal issues extended into adulthood, most likely not helped by Shackleton's struggle with alcohol dependence that plagued him throughout his life. While he believed that the warmth of a good woman was the only real cure for illness, after his first and second wife left him, he settled for a diet of grapes and managed to miraculously heal himself.

Grapes weren't the only fruit that naturopaths and alternative healers touted as miracle foods. On a mountain called Monte Verità on the border of Switzerland and Italy, a group of individuals created a colony based on the "ideal of a bloodless, vegetarian diet" where only fruit was to be eaten ("an Englishman who wanted fried potatoes had to leave"). The colony was sensationalized in some magazines; one article featured a photo of a fruit garden, a door with the statement "The Entrance to Paradise," and two members meant to evoke Adam and Eve "clad in skins," with the colony's owner presenting them with an apple. For some, this image made the colony seem like a bunch of communistic fruit-eaters with their heads in the clouds. But for Arnold Ehret, a man who had struggled his whole life with health issues, including a heart condition and Bright's Disease, it looked like a dream. He established a similar colony and had so many visitors that he "had to lock [his] house-door." Even while he was delivering the message of fruit as a cure to so many patients, he longed for more: a "blessed isle with sun and fruit, away from the throng of people," but the experiences of a man named August Engelhardt dissuaded him from leaving Switzerland for any island. Englehardt, Ehret writes, lived in the Bismarck Archipelago of Papua New Guinea and edited a journal called *Sun, Coconut, and Grapes.* While he had all the sustenance he might desire, he was desperate for company; not even his wife would live with him, and three men who traveled there to experience a life of endless fruit died not long after arrival. That didn't stop Englehardt from writing about his "happy life" there, and Ehret, though he never moved to an island, did continue to preach about the power food had over health, eventually writing *Professor Arnold Ehret's Mucusless Diet Healing System: Scientific Method of Eating Your Way to Health.*

* * *

It seems that anyone trying a fruit-based diet at that time couldn't help but spread the news, and *The Herald of the Golden Age* served as a central publication through which various practitioners dispensed their burgeoning knowledge. Readers of the *Herald* would have seen articles like the one published in 1909, "The Value of the Banana," which celebrated the "wonderful results" of physicians curing patients using "a banana-cure (i.e., dieting their patients exclusively on bananas until cured)" and claiming that bananas could help sedentary people stay healthy; nursing mothers yield more milk; small children grow stronger bones; and recommended bananas as a "splendid food" for people who might be diabetic, anemic, emaciated, or suffering from kidney trouble. Another article, "The Banana Cure," emphasized many of these same claims, while also noting that the banana could be used to "dress blistered wounds" and serve "as a rest for the eye in ophthalmia" or satisfy choleric thirst. In a deeply problematic colonial endnote to the article, the author suggests that the "country people" who have to do "rough work" are able to "be so powerful" because they are nourished by plantains.

Extending beyond bananas, various articles make cases again and again for how pure—and purifying—fruit is as a food source. Josiah Oldfield, for example, in rhetoric that sounds much like the crescendo of a sermon, writes, "With the right use of fruits for food what a glory of health results. I have seen the clogged and sluggish liver cleansed and purified to new life. I have seen the creeping consumption stayed in its dank pathway of death. I have seen the blotched and lepra skin come clean and like a child's again. Aye, and I have seen the hopeless pick up stray gleams of hope, and put a quavering foot forward towards Life and Courage once more." This near worship of fruit as a savior from not only health maladies but also from fears surrounding the "confinement" brought about by industrialization extended beyond the borders of England.

As Morris Krok, a South African publisher and fruitarian, writes in the introduction to a republished edition of German fruitarian Otto Abramowski's text, *Fruitarian Diet and Physical Rejuvenation*, he discovered the book because an elderly lady living in Pietermaritzburg, South Africa, donated all her Order of the Golden Age literature to him. He received recipe books, bound volumes of the *Herald*, and a copy of Abramowski's book, in which he writes about how "the fruit fast has provided a wonderful factor in purifying the blood and strengthening the healing powers of nature." I mention this not only to illustrate the ways that fruitarianism began to spread throughout the world through colonialism, but also to note that the Order's presence in South Africa was strong enough to make it likely that Cornelius may have encountered literature that potentially swayed him to give up his fervent belief in peanut oil and inspired him to swap it out for fruit. The ways that Essie is fixated on purity in her memoir (she believed that being "wrong in our habits" and eating "misplaced food" would lead to "disease symptoms," "suffering and pain," and went against the "Creator's will") mirror many of the claims made in books like Abramowski's and in the pages of the *Herald*. Cornelius's fruit experiment then might not have been such a brilliant stroke of isolated genius, as Essie suggests in her memoir, but more like soft plagiarism.

The dangers of guarding a certain kind of purity extended even further than the fruit diet itself. It is no coincidence that Arnold Ehret, Essie Honiball, Cornelius Valkenberg de Villiers Dreyer, Johanna Brandt, and company were all white. Lisa Betty, a PhD candidate in history at Fordham University, writes that Donald Watson coined the term "vegan" in 1944 when he founded The Vegan Society, which was "unequivocally colonial, white centered-supremacist, and elitist. Culturally, Eurocentric veganism required moral astuteness, restriction, vigilance, and shame. It was not liberatory, intersectional, radical, or decolonial." As Khushbu Shah writes in the essay "The Vegan Race Wars:

How the Mainstream Ignores Vegans of Color," veganism has existed in communities of color through Rastafarianism, Jainism, Buddhism, Hinduism, and in the Black Hebrew Israelite community long before it was coined and commodified by white people, but those histories have often been ignored by mainstream media and white vegan influencers.

The whiteness of veganism has produced insidious results in the present day. One is the use of racist language employed by People for the Ethical Treatment of Animals (PETA) and other vegan organizations. PETA, according to Tara Roeder, has relied "on the objectification of women and people of color or the employment of fatphobia in its campaigns against animal cruelty," and Betty adds that the organization "is still propagating award winning trauma porn campaigns that compare nonhuman animal confinement to U.S. chattel slavery of Black people—even in court cases against animal abuse the organization used the 13th amendment." In addition to this harmful language, deeper systemic issues have meant a confluence of harms. As Amirah Mercer writes in her longform essay "A Homecoming," food deserts disproportionately impact Black and Latino communities, and "systemic racism within the dietetics industry has kept Black dietitians out of the field—their number has fallen by nearly 20 percent over the last two decades." People of color have been systemically excluded from vegan organizations. Isaias Hernandez, on his blog *Queer Brown Vegan*, cites a study from 2005 showing that out of "the 32 animal welfare organizations featured in the study, 13 organizations were found not to have a single black employee. For the other 19 organizations, it was found that no more than 7% of the employees were black." Without an intersectional, intentional approach to dismantling these systems, they remain intact. As Hernandez writes, until people are willing to "interrogate their own white supremacy" and stop "ignoring the effects of colonization and how it is interconnected to the oppression of humans and animals," nothing meaningful will change.

White supremacy and certain strains of veganism have existed hand in hand since organizations like The Order of the Golden Age were founded. Because veganism is so sprawling, this book in no way captures all the harms—and joys—that different communities have found in this way of eating, nor does it chronicle in any meaningful way the histories of veganism in practice. Instead, I introduce this information because examining the unrelenting whiteness of vloggers and influencers associated with a high-carb, low-fat, raw vegan diet means studying the ways in which the racist origins of the idea of weight loss and wellness have influenced the present. Sabrina Strings writes that "the crux of the issue" is that "the image of fat black women as 'savage' and 'barbarous' in art, philosophy, and science, and as 'diseased' in medicine has been used to both degrade black women *and* discipline white women." That many of the prolific vegan YouTubers in the 2010s were white and that very few—if any—acknowledged the origins of veganism within communities of color, *and* that many embraced goals of weight loss or a thin "dream body," relates directly to the ways in which women's bodies have been surveilled, controlled, and shaped throughout history and into our present day.

*   *   *

On the fruit diet, as Essie grew stronger both physically and in her resolve to continue eating the way Cornelius commanded, she also developed more serious feelings for the man she believed had saved her from sickness. They married, and Essie writes that soon after, Cornelius "withdrew [her] from normal life." While this lack of agency on Essie's part, at least in the way the sentence in her book is crafted, might be alarming (especially paired with statements like Cornelius showing her "no mercy" and subjecting her to "relentless discipline"), the nature of their relationship continues to be murky. Several circumstances contribute to this. One is their large age gap; Essie was in her thirties and Cornelius was seventy-six. But more than that, Essie was pregnant with a different married man's child, and circumstances in South Africa at the time would mean that she could experience severe social ostracization, as well as professional consequences, if she let anyone know about it. Anoeschka von Meck, Essie's biographer, posits that Cornelius might have married Essie out of kindness more than passion; his marriage to her offered protection from the wider world. But Anoeshcka notes, too, that Essie had complicated, often codependent relationships with men throughout her life.

What I fear that I have done while writing Essie's story is treat it like Freelee and Durianrider would later treat food on their online platforms: flatten a nuanced narrative into good and bad, blood or fruit. Eating fruit and fruit alone is not the issue. Instead, the ways that the fruit cure has been evangelized, monetized, and weaponized is a symptom of something much larger, one that stretches back all the way to the racist origins of thinness itself.

The fruit diet holds the potential for harm—both in body and mind—but also for healing. Anoeschka told me about a moment so beautiful and mystical that she found it difficult to translate. "Many expressions in Afrikaans have such an atmosphere, so much color, that for me to put it in English feels like I'm going from technicolor to black and white." In the memory, as Anoeshka narrated to me, "It's early morning and [Tannie Essie]'s looking at the moon. The moon is like a piece of pumpkin. It's orange. And she's between fruit trees, barefoot. Even though she's in her eighties, she's like this fairy girl. She feels the wet blades of grass against her legs, and the whole garden has this atmosphere and the fireflies are moving between the trees. And she has three of them in her hand. Have you seen a firefly up close? She feels this presence. She's not alone. It is the Creator, the one that she calls the Beloved is with her. She's looking at these fireflies in her hand and she's letting them go, she's putting them back on a branch, and she's thinking, Beloved, is this how you hold starry planets in the palm of your hand, just little twinkling lights?"

When I think about Essie, I want to remember her this way—as a woman who, nearing the end of her life, still experienced wonder and found peace. There is no way of knowing what Essie and Cornelius's marriage might have been like, but it is clear he *did* care for her. Not long after Cornelius whisked the two of them away in a van, Essie delivered a stillborn baby, a traumatic event that haunted her throughout her life. However, that time period is one she also remembered as sweet. Essie spent each day sunning herself and eating fresh fruit right from the tree or vine. When she returned, her family and friends could hardly believe their eyes. Tan, stronger, and thoroughly rested, Essie felt "full of the joys of life."

CHAPTER 7

Sick

AT A FOLLOW-UP APPOINTMENT WITH THE NEUROLOGIST
near campus in early fall, I asked about my ability to complete a
marathon. The doctor told me to be mindful of any symptoms, but
to go for it. Aside from long periods of time spent on the elliptical
over the summer in Missouri and a few runs here and there, I had
not trained regularly since my farmland runs the previous fall. As
I charted out a training plan for myself, the familiar thrill of a new
season returned to me. Ahead of me unfurled months of hard work,
long stretches of miles on weekend mornings, aching legs, and a stamp
of sweat marking me as a runner again. My return to the sport was
humbling. In my initial days of training, four miles—which previously
would have been considered relief—left me gasping for breath. I kept
trying. I ran down the farmland roads as I had the previous year, this
time not for pain but in pursuit of something different. My head was
clear. My voice did not warble or break. My legs did not fail me. In
rare moments, with the sun warming my shoulders and the road wide
open and empty before me, I felt like I was suspended in a dance that
would never end.

At the end of October, I walked down a street in Washington, D.C. wearing a black trash bag over my clothing, the air cold enough that breath plumed from my mouth like smoke. Tens of thousands of other people moved in the same direction as me. I hopped from foot to foot, giddy. When I heard the crack of the gun, it echoed with a whole history of starts. The course took me up George Washington Parkway, across Key Bridge where I looked over the calm Potomac, along the cobblestone streets of Georgetown, and down long stretches where the monuments were visible on one side and cherry trees slumbered on the other. Thick crowds of people lined the course with signs and cowbells and speakers. From the wall of noise, I heard a familiar refrain, some music that had been quiet for years: My mom yelled "Go, Jack, go!" and my dad said, "C'mon, J-a-c-q-u-e, kick it! Kick it, turtle!" They had been there for me through illness, encouraging me over the phone and, when they could, flying out to see me, but it was hearing their voices that made my breath catch in my throat. For a moment, it felt like we had all made it to safety, to a place where I wouldn't fear falling any longer.

When I write this scene, part of me wishes I could end my story here, at this marathon. I could say: I overcame my symptoms, I returned to my sport, I was whole. Perhaps I did believe that if I ran a marathon, I would never have to worry again. If I ran a marathon, I could end my story with an image of me making my way up the last hill, my eyes filling with tears, my arms swinging strong. I could end with the weight of a medal around my neck, running to meet my parents, both of them effervescent. At the time, those endings were true. I crossed the finish line, happier than I'd been in a long time. I placed first in my age division. I trained without any flicker of an episode returning.

But it wasn't the end. Instead, two and a half months later, with approval from my neurologist, I traveled to Peru to study abroad for a three-week intersession. The trip is a blur. All I remember now is the towering, pale yellow facade of the Basílica Convento de San Francisco in Lima; colorful, wrought-iron balconies that overlooked bustling streets; waves beating against a rocky shore; the hush of museums; and the steep, vivid green of the Colca Canyon, a couple of condors weaving through blue sky above. When I look back now, everything is hazy, just out of reach. The exact moment of my body's failure escapes me. Was it when I was on my way to Spanish class in Arequipa? My legs straining uphill, the dull pressure settling in my brain. Street dissolving. Or was it later? On the bus? When I try to see the scene, it's as if low, strange clouds obscure my vision. I can scavenge fragments, not full cloth.

Here, sew them together: *the back of the bus seat had   royal blue,*
soft-sharp   jade green and mustard   fu c h s i a
confetti lines   head starts rocking—does it
?—and I press   forehead against
seat   brain clenched fist too tight and
pulsing   pain   dizzying sense of flight—I
am flying,   flying, I am spinning, put me down,
body holding me—   he says her head is spinning
does it usually   should I keep carrying her
head is spinning I dunno it's rocking on its own—silky cotton of
hotel   and

When I woke up, I was in a hotel room, enveloped by a pillowy white duvet. The low clouds of my early illness had returned. This time, they were here to stay.

*   *   *

A doctor visited me in the hotel room. In an echo of the athletic trainer's desire to quantify what was wrong, he took my blood pressure and pulse. He held the metal diaphragm of a stethoscope to my chest. My memory of this time is dim enough that I do not remember specific conversations or precise chronology. But I do remember explaining to the doctor and my professors that I had a neurological condition. The blurred vision, the loss of memory, the way my speech dissolved into repeated, sometimes slurred, words—all of it was familiar to me. The doctor told me that I was okay, except for altitude sickness. He explained that when I ate, blood was rushing from my brain to my stomach. He told me to refrain from consuming large amounts of food. He left. Someone brought me a large bottle filled with an electrolyte drink. I fell asleep.

When I woke up, the sun was near setting. I lay still and surveyed the room around me. Bedside table with a half-empty electrolyte drink. A window that looked out onto a darkening verdant courtyard. Crisp white duvet. I sat up in bed and my head echoed with that eerie pressure, the way a sky stills before a storm. If I moved, my vision grew blurry. Someone came in to check on me and brought a plate of spaghetti. I was hungry, but the image of blood rushing from my brain to my stomach, however flawed the prognosis might have been, was something for me to fixate on. I ate just two bites before setting the plate down and falling asleep again. I don't remember much after that—was I there for days? for hours in that bed?—but I remember that my classmates left for a day excursion and I declined to go. My professor asked to meet for lunch in the hotel's courtyard restaurant. I don't remember whether or not I told her that I wasn't well, that I could feel the symptoms rising in me like an unholy tide. My legs felt shaky, even during my careful steps to the bathroom, but I had to get to the restaurant. The stairs to get there were built from flat, smooth pieces of rock. The bright green of the world turned to a pinprick of dark. I collapsed. Someone found me. When I woke up, I was in bed again. Next to me, through the speaker of the hotel phone, was the sound of my mother's voice, my father's. The Dean. They decided, based on my condition, that it was best I return to campus immediately.

The days that followed exist to me only as choppy fragments: my professor leaving me alone in the airport so she could get a massage, a wheelchair ride down a long corridor in Miami, the cool air of a car, familiar strip malls and outlets near North Carolina's highway whizzing by, and then a room. A hotel bed. Curtains that kept the room dark even during the day. I slept. My mom put her hand against my forehead, the way she had when I was small. Those days are the sour-salt taste of Tom Yum broth, a dark room, sleep. My mom taking short walks with me, dissolving into haze. Sleep. The sound of her voice murmuring into a phone. Sleep. Gone was the girl who had crossed a marathon finish line. In her place was a patient who could not walk the length of a cul-de-sac without succumbing to dizziness and a slurred string of syllables. When my mom took me to the neurologist, he seemed more concerned than he had in the past. At a visit earlier that fall, as I discovered years after the fact, he had written, "Patient close to tears during this interview," as if to mark my symptoms as emotional rather than physical. But this time, he listed "CONVULSIONS" in all caps. He encouraged me to get on a waitlist at Duke University Hospital for a stay in the epilepsy monitoring unit. My mom and I both said yes.

Maybe my mom left when classes started for spring, or maybe she left because she had to get back home, I don't remember. I moved from the hotel bed to my apartment. I remember trying to take classes, but the words blurred away from me on the page, and even a short conversation left me ready to sleep for hours. In the past, I had pushed through moments of discomfort, walked to classes symptomatic, and tried to run even when there was a chance of collapse. This time around, it was physically impossible for me to make it through a full day of school without symptoms overtaking me. I finally sought the rest that I had avoided in previous years. I wanted to go home to where my parents lived, in Oklahoma, to elude the daily reminders that I was not living a normal life on campus. I wanted to be cared for. I remember calling my parents. The conversation that came next was one of the hardest in our relationship. My parents told me I should stay at school. I wept. I told them I wanted—needed—to come home. They said they had spoken with the Dean, who would allow me to drop every class but one for the purpose of staying on campus; my apartment was only an hour or so from the hospital where I'd undergo testing. At the time, I couldn't fully understand their decision; all I felt was hurt that I had finally reached out and been met with a decision that felt like my parents had not heard me. It is only in adulthood looking back that I realize things weren't so clear cut. The dance I had performed for years, pretending I was fine when I wasn't, had backfired. They wanted to keep me safe, and thought being in the apartment with my friends would make me happy. Because I did not tell them really anything that had happened to me—not the sexual assault, not suicidal ideation, not the taunting from my teammates, not what it felt like to live in fear that any moment an episode would snatch me from wherever I was trying to be—they were left to imagine what I had endured based on my behavior during brief visits at home, during which time I'd tried to conceal mercurial bouts of anger, sadness, and despondency. Though I had only shown my parents the scars of my depression and not the depths, they lived in a constant state of fear when the phone rang. They have ghosts that haunt them from those years, too.

My parents gave me money for a wheelchair, and I chose a cherry red one with a cup holder. It was a travel chair, which meant someone had to push me around. Without school to attend each day, without the physical ability to leave my room, and without anyone around the apartment for most of every day, I was, for the first time, really alone. I had a blue papasan chair in my bedroom, and I spent most of my days there. I cried more than I ever have in my life. At the time, I couldn't understand the severity of my sadness. Or maybe I was too tired to trace its contours. But now, looking back, I see that I felt trapped between impossibilities.

Because the symptoms had receded after I left the team, a team-mate's voice had stayed with me, taunting, "You're faking all of this, you freak." My illness, in some moments, had felt real while I was on the team: There was an assistant coach to carry me to the training room. There were teammates who bore witness to my head rocking in circles in the dining hall. There were video clips of the aphasic strings of words that came from my mouth. But while I could find proof of sickness in my body's failings, in the way that symptoms overtook me, I also felt pressed against a wall of disbelief. In the eyes of the athletic doctor, the trainer, my coach, the neurologist, and all the other medical professionals I had seen—the MRI tech, the cardiologist, the ophthal-mologist—nothing was wrong with me. I was normal. Well developed. Capable of running a marathon if I wanted. No sign of seizures or any other abnormalities detected. As Susan Wendell, a feminist disability theorist, writes, when patients who express symptoms are disbelieved or when their symptoms are not validated or confirmed by medical authorities, they can turn doubt on themselves rather than questioning the care of doctors. "Medicine can undermine our belief in ourselves as knowers, since it can cast authoritative doubt on some of our most powerful, immediate experiences," she writes. "Moreover, the power of medicine also subjects us to possible private and public invalidation by others—invalidation as knowers and as truth-tellers."

In the two years that had passed since I first collapsed and quit the team, I had lived in a liminal space between believing in my illness and pretending nothing was wrong with me. My motto was, basically: if the doctors—trained neurologists—say I'm okay, I must be; if Coach and my teammates insinuate it's all in my head, it must be. A lack of confir-mation from medical professionals for years had led me to question my own reality, to undermine the inklings of symptoms that tugged at me from time to time. But when I returned from Peru, I felt my carefully constructed lies of *I'm fine* crashing down around me. Sitting in my apartment alone day after day, I could no longer live in a half-fictional reality. I had no choice but to experience my body again, to recognize the symptoms I had tried to pretend did not exist.

Here, stand up and let your body sway a little, like a tulip in a strong spring wind. Roll your head gently in circles, as if warming up for an event you won't compete in. Open a book, blur your vision, and sit there staring at what used to be words. Wake up in your papasan chair. Blink, as if that might bring back your memory. Look at the way the dust motes swirl in the late afternoon light. Wonder where the day went. Pretend you don't mind not knowing. Do it all alone. Tell no one. And when your roommates come home, bringing that blessed cacophony of backpacks thudding against carpet and keys jangling and stories from days spent outside, emerge from your room and try your best to scrounge up something—anything—you did in the hours they were gone.

*   *   *

Even now, as I relive those memories, I have a hard time doing it in first person, reminding myself: I experienced this. I felt my vision blur. My head rocked, unwillingly. I lived through unremembered hours, with no one to keep record of what happened to me or my body when I slipped away. I felt helpless. When I think back to that time period, a current of shame and fear runs through me. Shame for the ways I couldn't wrangle my body into submission. During my months of initial visits with the neurologist, he told me to keep an Excel sheet chronicling what I ate each day, barometric pressure, hours I had slept, and stress levels, as well as whether or not I was episodic. All of life's uncertainties categorized neatly within the rows of a spreadsheet. I should have loved it the way I loved graphing Halloween candy by type when I was a kid, organizing the colorful chaos on the living room carpet, or keeping years' worth of running statistics in a binder organized by date, each mile split written out by hand. But I didn't. Instead of identifying a pattern, I found no certain reason for my symptoms. Some days when I was episodic there was stress, some days I ate a bowl of Quaker Oatmeal Squares and wondered if they were the cause, some days I'd try to find meaning in low grey clouds outside or convince myself I hadn't slept enough. My whole life, through sport, I had learned to equate control with power, with praise. The more I could suppress my own bodily instincts, the more I could quiet those murmurs of soreness or discomfort, the better I was. But there, sitting in my chair, my inability to overcome was laid bare.

I was afraid, at that time, of never getting better. In the past, there had been periods of release, moments where my head cleared. This time was different. As days passed, my radius of orbit stayed the same: bed, chair, bathroom, chair, kitchen, chair. I grew deeply angry with my body for failing me, and angry with myself for somehow failing my body. I had laid as still as a rabbit beneath the mechanical whir of the MRI machine, submitted my veins time and time again for whatever needed to be taken, allowed my body to be tilted, scanned, tested, prodded, measured, and described. None of it had led to clarity, and for that I felt responsible. I hadn't eaten well enough, visited the doctor enough, prayed hard enough. I had run too hard, gone to altitude. I wasn't as strong as someone else might be in my position. If I were Coach, I'd have found a way to rise out of my chair, ace my classes, and remain on the team, making all of it look effortless. I'm now aware that I am not so alone in this feeling. Susan Wendell writes that because of our collective refusal to face the "realities of bodily life," individuals who are disabled or ill carry the burden of finding a treatment for themselves.

During those long days spent alone in my room, my desk became an altar, Google a god I prayed to: *Am I epileptic?* (*I want to walk again.*)

Am I sick? (I am afraid.) And the internet responded with quizzes to tell me whether or not I had temporal lobe epilepsy, infographics with symptoms of a stroke, advice on whether to exercise with seizures. I took every test to see whether or not I could determine what was wrong with me. I read stories of people who had suddenly fallen ill. I tried to find myself in a variety of WebMD descriptors that became a funhouse mirror for my own symptoms.

When I had exhausted all that, I clicked on a website that would change everything: I found the two banana-wielding gurus I thought might be able to save me.

CHAPTER 8

Testify

WITHIN THE BIBLICAL GARDEN OF EDEN, THERE ARE TWO notable trees: one of life, and one that holds the knowledge of good and evil. God instructs Adam, then a nameless man, that he may "eat freely of every tree of the garden; but of the tree of the knowledge of good and evil you shall not eat, for in the day that you eat of it you shall die." God is omniscient; the man, new. Scholars, when analyzing this moment in the text, propose that this might have been a time when man—and later woman—had access to immortality. What if Eve had eaten from the tree of life and ignored the tree of good and evil? What did her curiosity cost?

I imagine Adam and Eve wandering the garden in bodies that were at once natural to them and entirely mysterious. If thinking about them as humans, fallible and without God's omniscience, I imagine that there must have been fear running alongside their wonder. What foods might sustain them? Why, if paradise was truly paradise, would the nectar of any fruit be off-limits? So often, Eve is characterized nega-tively as being tempted by the fruit, but considering how Eve must have felt when the snake first whispered sweet promises in her ear, I see her thirst for knowledge. A curiosity about her own body and the world. Who wouldn't want a taste? When I think about that moment in the garden, I see myself sitting before my laptop, begging for something that would help me better know myself. I see Essie, tripping over a hose at the pool, wondering if she would ever swim again. I see all of us who, impacted by illness and exhaustion and age, might, if we could, reach for something forbidden that would teach us how best to live.

When my browser first loaded, the *30 Bananas a Day* (30BaD) website populated with a faded header of spotty bananas, an advertisement for "The Woodstock Fruit Festival," and a smiling apple parachuting from the sky toward a dancing cucumber. There were people with usernames like The FruitMonster, HunnyDew Sunshine, BeeFree, and Ivegonebananas. They left comments on forums titled:

Fresh Dates! How long do they last??
VEGANS! Do you compare animal life worth to human life worth?
Ah! What am I to do??? My fiance is anti-vegan!
I'm scared to eat.
Hi, newbie questions incoming
Are meals of carrots ok?
Terribly itchy legs at night, please help :(
Fruit stops sickness?

I'll admit, I laughed. Whether it was the unaesthetic bright green and pale yellow borders outlining forums or phrases like "high vibe community!," "30BaD Peacekeepers," and "fruit-munchers" used in earnest, the site seemed at first like something funny to share with my roommates when they got home, something that would allow me to add my voice to the chorus of their days. Two of my roommates-turned-best-friends, Eliza and Andrea, were vegan at the time, so I was well aware of what that meant: no meat, no eggs, no animal products of any kind, honey included. They had both been vegan before moving in and were respectful, if not fervent, when they spoke about their beliefs. (It probably helped that during those years I was too intimidated to try cooking meat on my own, so I ate what we jokingly termed a "gorilla vegan diet," as I shared 98% of their eating habits.)

I never became fully vegan in the years that I lived with them, but I was jealous of their certainty. They watched documentaries like *Forks Over Knives* and used the footage as fuel for the way they felt about the world. Around Thanksgiving, they ranted about the conditions in which turkeys were kept; in captivity, unable to run around, the poultry developed bodies that were too heavy for their legs. In their journey with veganism at the time, there did not seem to be room for nuance or exception; their commitment was so strong that I still Google the ingredients of red food dye to see if it includes Red 40 (a petroleum byproduct that technically is fine to eat but some vigilant vegans avoid because it has been tested on animals) and ask vegan friends if they mind which brand of white sugar I use before I bake for them (in our college apartment, we only used organic white sugar from the co-op because other sugar might have been processed through animal bone char).

While I felt—and still feel—empathy for the animals, food was more complicated to me. (Even now, as I write this sentence, I hear echoes of vegans on the internet telling me that if I *truly* cared, it would not be complicated at all.) I enjoyed sharing meals with my roommates and was grateful to learn more about their lifestyle, but I found it difficult to hold such a hard line in my own life in determining the "right" way of eating from "wrong." I found too much joy in a bowl of my grandma's homemade chicken noodle soup, for example. My grandma used a recipe passed down from my great-great-grandma for the egg noodles and used a knife my grandpa had been gifted after working night shifts at a chicken place while my mom was growing up. I couldn't imagine believing something about food enough to turn down any of her cooking, so much of it steeped in history, labor, and love.

It was the same lack of certitude that had led me to fall away from formal religion after a lifetime of being brought up in the church; there was just something in me that had a hard time condensing the messiness of the world into a pinprick of something tangible I could trust. It wasn't that I didn't want to believe—in fact, I very much did. I wanted to belong to something greater than myself, to lose myself to the current of what I knew was right. One of the parallels between organized religion and veganism, at least in my experience, is that a believer in either has the tendency to think that their way of life is best, on a level of morality. To not believe—in God or veganism—means that you need saving or need to wake up to the harsh realities of what your life without belief is costing you. I wanted to be all in. I craved the safety of knowing, definitively, that I was "good," but I had too many questions. How was locally raised meat bad but fruit flown all the way across the world any better, on an environmental level? What about people who couldn't access all the substitutes and specialty ingredients that we bought at the co-op each week?

I liked the freedom of eating a mostly vegan diet in college while still leaving room for spontaneity, cravings, or special moments with family. I wasn't against any diet, but I wasn't for any diet either, which I guess made me just curious enough. I became a sponge for rhetoric that was an echo of my own innermost thoughts. What I hoped to hear, at that time, was a way of making order from the chaos in my own life. The more time I spent on 30BaD, the more I realized it was unlike the veganism that I knew through my roommates—their veganism included cinnamon rolls slathered in vegan cream cheese, pizza from Mellow Mushroom covered with a thick layer of half-melted Daiya shreds, and chocolate chip cookie dough made with flax eggs. 30BaD was different. It offered me answers that would lift me from my loneliness and sickness.

Freelee and Durianrider, the founders, enlisted someone with the username PK (whose bio stated that they had a college degree in healthcare management, performed "Peacekeeping maneuvers" on the 30BaD website, and were qualified to "assist with patient education" based on their basic knowledge of human anatomy) to sum up the rules of the diet for the public. "In a banana peel," the diet was simple: Practitioners should eat fruits, lettuce greens, and a handful of nuts. The fruits should be raw, whole, and fresh. Women should consume 2,500 calories and men should eat 3,000. Followers should sleep eight to twelve hours per night and drink enough water to ensure their urine was always clear. If followers adhered to the rules, they were promised perfect health, clear skin, endurance, community, and more. They could heal themselves from ailments that had plagued them for years. Freelee and Durianrider wanted "low fat raw vegan lifestylists' and aspiring rawfoodies" to participate in the forums. The pair, who had fallen in love with raw fruit and with each other, wanted to "guard against the temptation to create a vision that is too broad" in order to yield more "fruitful results."

* * *

Their vision attracted people from around the world. Members joined from Sweden, the United Kingdom, Northern Ireland, Austria, Germany, Canada, Turkey, Belgium, New Zealand, Romania—name a place and there most likely was a 30BaD member who lived nearby. As I scrolled, I wondered: How had other people found the website? Did they seriously believe in the power of fruit, or were they like me, just lurking in wait for some kind of cure? From reading profiles, I learned that one member was "brought here by a YouTube video." Another joined the website after seeing her father-in-law "fight his stage 4 lung cancer with a vegan diet, superdoses of vitamins, and other natural methods." Community members came to the site to heal, because they believed that fruit was what God intended humans to eat, to save themselves from cancer, to stay thin, to lose weight, to rid themselves of acne, and to get in shape. One member, Raini Pachak, came to the diet because of a psychedelic experience he had in his best friend's basement when he was sixteen.

Growing up, Raini was a self-described typical skater kid. He ate a lot of junk food and smoked a lot of weed. At sixteen, while tripping on mushrooms, he "went to this space of understanding" where he realized he wanted to live in nature rather than society. He thought about how humans can be so backward, how everything we create is trash. "The city is litter" became one of his mantras. While tripping, he realized something that would change his life forever: The closer we get to nature, the healthier we can be. He thought about chimpanzees. What do they eat? Fruits and greens. When he came down from his high, he felt like he had been reborn. He didn't want to lose the meditative state he had experienced on the 'shrooms, so he stopped talking for the most part. He started eating fruits and greens, figuring he would stop if he didn't feel well. Some of his experience was positive; he had found a new diet that made him feel and look his best. Other parts of his experience limited his life for a while. For example, he began to believe that laughter is just something people do to please each other rather than a genuine, shared reaction. He resisted relationships, believing that true happiness would be found on his own, in nature. He didn't articulate his beliefs, as he didn't know how to at the time. This left his family and friends wondering what had happened to him and what he was feeling.

Raini solidified his calling to veganism while out in nature alone. He went out to a desolate area by himself, the closest he could get to really leaving society at seventeen, and slept there. He realized he should learn to talk again to spread his message: We could all live peaceful and enjoyable lives if only we reached toward what is good and true. So on his eighteenth birthday, he had a cup of coffee (which made him anxious, as he hadn't had caffeine in a long time) and asked his mom to drop him off at OfficeMax. He went inside, bought a marker and poster board, and wrote "YOU ARE NAKED" and "THE CITY IS LITTER." He held his poster up on the side of a busy road and meditated. It was "totally transcendental," Raini told me in a 2021 interview over Zoom. Raini felt like he was falling backward, "Like you're falling asleep and you've lost your posture." But when Raini opened his eyes, he was sitting upright. And when he looked up, "there was this freakin' orb, silver, mirror-finished like a silver chrome ball in the sky. It was big, probably the size of two or three cars put together. I just looked at it for a while and took it as a sign that I should be doing this. I took it as a sign that I am here, where I should be." He meditated for a while longer and was interrupted by his best friend, who asked, "What the fuck are you doing, Raini?" Raini got up and the two of them "went, like, rock climbing after that or something."

For the first three years after his psychedelic experience, Raini was a hardcore raw vegan, but, unlike Durianrider and Freelee, he ate fat. The bulk of his diet was salad, nuts, greens, and juices. He dropped his old friends, who were too into weed and junk food, and started hanging out at a raw food restaurant. As an alternative to college, Raini found WWOOFing (Worldwide Opportunities on Organic Farms), which took him to Uruguay. There, with a friend who was also vegan, he started eating cooked foods out of convenience. Immediately, Raini felt terrible. His skin itched, he couldn't sleep, and his body felt perpetually inflamed and uncomfortable. The cooked food, for him, was a stepping stone to his old lifestyle; he started smoking weed again. It was around the time he turned twenty, three-ish years after he first went vegan, that he found 30BaD. In his profile picture on the site, he's wearing a bright red baseball cap slightly askew and a set of black headphones. He's smiling, and his nose and cheekbones are brushed pink from time in the sun. Behind him, a wall of periwinkle clouds part to let the bright white light of the sun shine through. His profile lists his location as Salt Lake City, Utah. As a response to the question, "Please tell us more about yourself and what brought you to the Frugivore Diet," Raini wrote, "I am what i do, i am what i eat. I am it, it is me." His gender is listed as "hunk," his favorite "book is a work in progress," and favorite "movie will end as i exhale, for the last time."

"I met cool people on *30 Bananas a Day*," Raini told me. Back in the day, 30BaD helped him find other people who ate the same way he did and offered a space where he could access helpful resources. On the site, he met someone who lived in Sedona, Arizona, who let him live with her as part of a work trade for six months. He liked the information that the moderators provided. While Raini would eventually feel that "Harley and Freelee let their fame get the best of them," in the beginning, he considered Freelee and Durianrider to be "really good influences. They seemed like good people."

* * *

The semester I found 30BaD, Eliza, who had been my confidante and a tether to a world I sometimes struggled to see myself in, was studying abroad. I had reverted to my old habit of withholding information so she wouldn't worry about me while she was gone. In her absence, Andrea did all she could to care for me. We laughed a lot—Andrea once spontaneously donned a sparkly leotard in our living room and attempted (without any formal gymnastics training) to recreate a routine she had seen at the Olympic games. We shared dinners, watched bad reality TV, and had a routine every night where we would put on matching waffle shirts so baggy they reached mid-thigh before we retreated to our separate rooms. Even with Andrea's friendship, I felt a great deal of loneliness that semester. There were so many hours that passed when she was in class or at a meeting for a club or just being a normal college student that I spent feeling like I was growing further and further behind. I couldn't exactly go out and meet new people, nor did I particularly want to in the precarious state of health that I was in;

the memories from the team were still too fresh for me to trust people outside my apartment.

Consequently, I had a lot of free time, stuck in my room, and more than anything, I was drawn to the glow of my screen. While I'm sure I must have visited other websites, 30BaD became a fixture of my daily routine. Sometimes I visited because the absurdity made my own reality seem more normal (like a list of "Frequently Asked Questions" posted by Freelee that suggests if you crave eating "animal poo" or your "attitude starts to suck" it means you aren't getting enough calories from fruit). Sometimes the website was a salve for solitude, and other times a form of escape. And sometimes, it moved me in a meaningful way, one I didn't yet have words for. From reading through forums, it seemed to me that most of the followers had suffered something significant in their past—they were trying to rid themselves of illnesses that had gone undiagnosed for years, addressing eating disorders, or resolving symptoms they no longer wanted to manage with medication. I found people who echoed my own deepest pain. I found rules that promised me what medical professionals couldn't. Like me, people who clicked on the website seemed at a loss for other options; they had exhausted all the possibilities that made sense. Unlike me, they had found an answer. They had left their old, sick selves behind and had returned to their former radiance.

They all posted about their miraculous recoveries on a page called "Testify!" In 2012, when I was frequently visiting the site, the page's header featured a pair of cartoon bodybuilders holding up a weightlifting bar stacked with plates. The man had a six-pack, bulging biceps, and a Speedo that showed off the strength of his quads. The woman, in a barely there black bikini, was equally jacked. She held her hand in a thumbs-up sign while the man curled a giant brown duffel bag marked "BANANAS," the spotty yellow ends of bananas spilling out the sides. This, the image seems to say, is who you could be if you just picked up fruit at the supermarket—an emblem of strength, smiling, part of a community. And the testimonials were equally overt in their messaging. As I scrolled, I saw my deepest desires laid bare:

> Comment by Shannana Bannana on July 3, 2011 at 8:18 am
>
> I am so grateful I found 30 BAD and the LFRV life!!!!!...I was a professional athlete (rower) training 4-6 hours per day and on the paleo diet. (side-note I am a 24 year old female, 5'10" as a rower I was 170 lbs and 18% body fat). After being severely over-trained I was diagnosed with adrenal fatigue, hoshimoto's, leaky gut, exhausted immune system, stress fractures in my back/ribs, and weight gain. In desperation I followed multiple doctors through excruciating and embarrassing tests, detox's, and weight loss plans. Then I hit a wall - I couldn't go on and that day I went 80/10/10 High carb, low fat/protein, raw vegan. Which was a complete 180 from the high protein, high fat, low carb diet I was on before. I have never felt better!!! Now I have so much energy!!! I'm training again, this time in running, I am teaching yoga classes, I am emotionally and physically balanced.

I didn't know Shannana Bannana, but it felt like she knew me—she had lost her life as an athlete, been put through the wringer by doctors to no avail, and finally felt good. I wanted what she now had—not only my health, but to feel like I was well in other ways. I wanted to finish my undergraduate degree. Feel tender toward my body again. See friends outside of the apartment. Experience gratitude rather than grief. Shannana Bannana, through her testimony, offered a way forward. So did others who had loaded up their banana wagons and started the diet. Scrolling down the pages and pages of different people's testimonies was like riding a carousel of fruit-filled positivity: My skin is clear! I'm rarely bloated! I was able to give up nearly all supplements! Life is beautiful! My confidence has soared! I don't have an ounce of cellulite on my body! I'm sooo hydrated and drinking so much water I can't help but be happy! I owe Douglas Graham my life! I now experience soaring energy! I know that I've found THE ANSWER!

I wanted nothing more than THE ANSWER. The answer would mean I could get out of my travel chair—in a moment as miraculous as a biblical tale—and walk around again. The answer would mean I'd have a body I'd want to flaunt. I might be able to cancel my appointment in the epilepsy unit and explain it all away as some big misunderstanding, just an imbalance in my nutrition. I might be able to eradicate the toxins in me, the darkness that seemed to swell up out of nowhere. Because of my own disgust with my symptoms, my own frustration with the lack of tangible answers from doctors over the years, and the messages about how my body should look at its most desirable that had been baked in since birth, I wasn't a difficult sell. When Freelee posted a montage video on her YouTube channel set to "beats by Danny Kirsch," featuring a series of pictures of her looking glum with phrases like, "I had enough. It was time to take control of my life," I thought, *I want that, too.* When her body transformed in photographs—she's flexing! Her skin is clear! She's eating half of a watermelon; the abundance! She cycled across all of Australia! In forty days!—to the sound of trumpets, the synthetic beat rising to a euphoric pitch, I thought, *I want that, too. Transform me. Set the footage of my life to the sound of exultant brass.* To get the life that Freelee had, all I had to do, according to a text slide in her video, was eat "the right kind of food." Thankfully, 30BaD made it very clear what that meant.

If I imagine 30BaD as a kind of Eden, the garden is full of fruit, lettuce, and more fruit. Almost everything else is forbidden. No cheat days, no sick days. No garlic, salt of any origin, chlorella, chili pepper, agave, maca, liquid aminos, nutritional yeast, or gourmet raw dishes. No starchy foods allowed, as starches need to be cooked and heating food destroys nutrients, so why bother? (In a dazzling display of mental gymnastics, on the "30BaD Banana Wagon Tour," PK the moderator writes that potatoes don't contain vitamin C and, as humans can get scurvy without vitamin C, eating potatoes might cause gum disease and skin hemorrhages.) The instructions continue: Eat as little fat as possible. And, because of members experiencing symptoms like "indigestion, sour and or acidic stomach, acid reflux, blood sugar spikes, dizziness and brain fog, diarrhea, constipation," and more after drinking fruit juices, no juicing allowed. Beyond the diet itself, there were even more rules. PK playfully frames them as "Banana Peels: Please Avoid Slipping!" but beneath the punny exterior, the commandments are disconcerting. The rules include things like: We don't slip up on calorie restriction; we don't talk about alcohol, drugs, or weed; we don't eat too much fat; we don't use profanity; and we don't bash or question veganism as a lifestyle.

In an animated graphic at the end of the "Wagon Tour," a red stick figure slips on a banana peel and lands on their back. A yellow stick figure emerges from the background, offers a hand, and helps the red stick figure up. They hold hands and then the red stick figure bends over to pick the banana peel up from the ground. The peel soars above them, leaving a rainbow of pears, peaches, lemons, grapes, cherries, apples, and more in its wake. And from the rainbow, the stick figures pick fruits, eat them, and disappear together into a bright horizon holding hands. The messaging is elementary but clear: Slip up on the diet and you will literally fall. Fruit is the way and the life, a bright rainbow that brings compassionate people together. Stay with the group and your life will be better. A similar philosophy of belonging exists on the 30BaD website as it did in Eden: Follow the rules, and God—or the gods of the diet—will accept you and allow you to remain part of their community; break one, and you'll be punished. In the case of 30BaD, punishment could range from posts being removed to your account suspended, or worse, your health declining because you didn't follow the commandments.

Now, with the benefit of years of hindsight and the worst of my symptoms in the rearview mirror, this messaging reads as harmful. But when you are in the throes of illness, at least in my experience, there is something comforting about distilling the world into dichotomies: sick or well, bad or good, off-limits or completely nutritious. When so much seems unknowable about the very body you live in, it feels nice to stand on a firm platform made from rights rather than wrongs, even if the very platform itself is a false reality. At my most desperate, I didn't spend much time parsing through the rhetoric of the website or thinking about the larger systems at play. Instead, compared to the language in doctors' reports that had twisted the animal of my body into clinical coldness, I found relief in people like me sharing their symptoms openly online. Their tales of triumph looked close enough to my own desire that I felt a sense of release. Someone out there knew how I was feeling. As I visited the site day after day, the stick figures and emoji fruit began to look less like caricatures and more like relief.

Durianrider's YouTube channels, as well as the copious amount of drama surrounding the pair (such as "a baffling campaign for mass vasectomies and a secretive breakup that's spiraled into accusations of domestic violence"). We'll get to all that later, I promise, as the drama is part of who Freelee and Durianrider have shaped themselves to be. Their antics are a commodity. For as long as they've been on the internet, Freelee and Durianrider's monetary success and cultural relevance has relied, in large part, on their clickability and how many people consume their videos.

It makes sense, then, that in the mid-2010s, when Freelee and Durianrider were peaking as cultural figures, outlets portrayed the couple's content as "a rich tapestry of juvenile insanity" and the diet itself as "monkey business," "bananas," and "insane." The language matches the outrageousness of some of the unverified health claims made in Freelee and Durianrider's videos. To take the diet seriously would be its own kind of dangerous, but the way outlets like *Cosmopolitan* covered it, with an article titled "This Insane Instagram Diet Involves Eating 30 Bananas a Day: Which is just, well, bananas" seems unhelpful as well. The word "insane" seems to be just as much clickbait as Freelee's follow-up video: "Cosmo Mag calls my diet INSANE!!" Coupled with the portrayal of the diet as an "Instagram diet," as if the way of eating simply appeared in a well-curated square overnight; the real-world implications of people eating only fruit for years after embedding themselves in Freelee and Durianrider's online community remain elusive. The article denounces the diet as "severely flawed," "unhealthy," and "not a regiment [sic] you can stick to long-term," but doesn't go beyond that. What about the people who *did* commit to it long term? What about the people who saw the diet not as "insane" but as a source of hope? Sure, the rules of the diet were (and are) ridiculous, and sure, you would probably be hard-pressed to find a credible dietitian who would recommend a steady stream of blended bananas as a long-term plan, and sure, the diet might count under the category of a "fad," but reducing it in these ways means not taking the time to understand how the diet came to be, the surprisingly relatable background of the couple who brought it to the forefront of vegan YouTube, and the followers who got swept up in the movement not because of "insanity" but because of a kind of deep longing that most of us have felt at one time or another.

In 2015, at the height of 30BaD's popularity, 28,130 people had created accounts on the site and 382,923 subscribed to Freelee's YouTube account (her personal YouTube following rose to 789,311 by July 2019, though the 30BaD website numbers stagnated). In early spring of 2012, when I found 30BaD, just 9,823 people were using the site, and the couple's only engagement with the press was through websites like Fruit-Powered.com (read: a very small platform compared to an outlet like *Cosmo*) where Freelee was sharing tips like "Proper food combining is 'absofruitly' essential for looking and feeling my best" and "If I get consistently undercarbed or undereat, the 'biatch' emerges."

I don't include this information to sound like some hipster saying, "I knew them before they were cool," but to set the stage a little more clearly. When I first encountered Freelee and Durianrider, they had no real mainstream mentions or presence, so they seemed, in a way, harmless. Or at least if not harmless, they seemed more like me than they do now. Less "guru profiting from views" and more "quirky friend who's got a weird trick that might help you heal."

When writing this book, I wanted to include Leanne and Harley's perspectives. I reached out to Harley via email, and he sent me a response within two hours saying, "Sure, I'd be happy to chat. Ask me ANY questions. Nothing is off topic for me." However, he did not respond to multiple follow-up emails I sent about scheduling an interview, or to subsequent emails that included a list of questions specifically related to claims I've made in the following pages. I reached out to Leanne multiple times through the contact form on her website, the email address associated with her public YouTube account, and through direct message on Instagram, and sent her multiple copies of questions specifically related to claims I've made in the following pages but did not receive any response from her. As a result, part of me feels—and will probably always feel—like I don't fully know Leanne and Harley, whose stories hold far more nuance and depth than the profiles they have curated online.

While there are surely gaps between their real, lived lives and the wealth of material posted publicly to YouTube, Instagram, and more, Leanne and Harley—as Freelee and Durianrider—have crafted a very public narrative over the past decade. They have interviewed each other about eating habits. They have divulged their thoughts about other influencers, about veganism, about each other, about themselves. They have filmed banal moments and momentous ones. I don't mistake any of this for closeness, not usually. I am too aware that these videos have been filmed, edited, and uploaded. I am seeing reality filtered through a screen and a lens. There has come a point, though, after reading all their e-books and watching a large portion of a decade's worth of footage, that I feel like I *do* recognize parts of them, maybe because in seeing them, I see parts of myself. Underneath their online antics are just two people who were once as desperate and depressed as I was ten years ago. When I glimpse that side of them, Freelee and Durianrider look less like all-knowing gods in a garden, and more like Adam and Eve—two humans who tried living up to unrealistic expectations and stumbled in paradise.

Before Freelee found her way to bananas, before she lost forty pounds, before she evolved into a self-proclaimed "Author, International speaker and educator, YouTube health guru, online raw food coach, and all round fit bitch," and before she turned venomous online toward anyone who disagreed with her teachings, Freelee was a child who was raised on a farm in Queensland, Australia. Her name was Leanne. In a photo of Leanne as a child, featured in her e-book *Go Fruit Yourself,* she's wearing what looks like a beige raincoat or an oversized button-down, a white cotton T-shirt beneath, blonde hair reaching just past her shoulders. A bird roosts in the crook of one of her outstretched arms and another is perched atop her taupe bucket hat. Leanne's face is wide open with a smile. On the farm, Leanne's family tended to a garden that yielded a bounty of produce, providing them with sweetness and nourishment. A cow named Missy was so patient that Leanne could drape herself across her back while Missy fed, the two of them soaking up sun. When Missy had a calf, Leanne and the baby played like a pair of puppies, chasing each other across the field and gently butting heads.

Though perhaps there were idyllic elements of this upbringing, Leanne's contemporary beliefs have rotted her perceptions of the past. Chickens remind her of abuse and slaughter. When she remembers Missy and her baby, she can only visualize calves stripped from their mothers and being "permanently confined to a box in which they cannot ever turn," the lack of movement keeping them tender. She thinks about what it would be like for humans to crawl into a field where a calf is nursing from their mother, "rip the calf away from her nipple," and attempt to suckle, procuring milk in its purest form rather than sanitized and commercially presented at the supermarket. In one of her e-books, Freelee writes, "When we consume milk products from ANY mammals (especially as females), we initiate the rape, exploitation and death of other female animals."

Freelee uses the word "rape" to characterize her childhood visits to the dentist, too; her teeth were "raped" of their innocence, she says, when about five of them were drilled for fillings. The cavities, she claimed, were caused not by sugar, but her lack of it. Even though the family garden produced plenty of fruit, Leanne was only allowed a couple pieces a day, per food pyramid guidelines. Leanne says now that she was "undercarbed," as most children are. Some days, to get more sugar she stole money to buy candy. Others, she hid in the food pantry, where she secretly mixed half a cup of powdered sugar with the sweet seeds of a passionfruit, eating it all in one sitting. For dinner most nights, her parents served fish, which she hated enough that she would hold a napkin in her hand, wait until her father was looking down at his own plate, spit up bite after bite, and stuff it into her pockets, flushing the meat down the toilet when she got the chance.

*   *   *

Search "Durianrider" on Google and your screen might populate with message boards discussing his athletic performances or public persona; websites like "The Ugly Truth About Harley 'Durianrider' Johnstone"; articles like "A Year of Bananas, Vasectomies, and Rape Allegations With the Vegans of YouTube"; and language like "controversial," "EXPOSED," "radical," and "vigilante" sprinkled throughout.

On his public Instagram, there is a video of his current girlfriend, Natasha, straddling the seat of her bike in the middle of a public sidewalk. She's wearing a pink helmet, low-cut bikini top or bra, and white bikini bottoms. The sound of Durianrider circling her with the camera, bike shoes scratching against the concrete, makes the video feel stilted. His caption is: "What 178 cm @61kg looks like. The best investment a girl can make is doing my protocols so she enhances/preserves her life freedom, health, aesthetics, relationships, hormones, finances and mental/physical performance." In another, his girlfriend is wearing a white crop top, white heels, and is leaning with her hand pressed against a white wall, looking back over her shoulder toward the camera. The thin strap of her white thong arches over her hip bone, revealing her bare butt. "Natasha bought my ebook when she was 17," Durianrider writes. "My protocols GUARANTEE you will get a stripper body! GUARANTEED!!" In his self-published e-book, Durianrider claims that you can beat depression by drinking water and "HTFU. If you don't know what this means. Google it." (Spoiler: it means "harden the fuck up.") On his Tumblr, when asked, "Can you cite any successes as a cyclist or runner?" he responds, "Why you such a fucking keyboard warrior but IRL you are such a pussy? . . .

What happened in your life that made you such a pussy keyboard warrior? FIGHT ME YOU PUSSY!"

Durianrider's online presence often strikes me as being vitriolic and misogynistic, and his messaging often repels me rather than encouraging me to draw near. But Durianrider was once a child named Harley Johnstone, and Harley Johnstone, at the age of eight, lay in a hospital bed. He felt like he was dying. In an interview published in 2009, Harley lists his health conditions, including "chronic fatigue, asthma, Crohn's disease, hypoglycemia, mild arthritis, sleep disorders, depression, drug addiction, alcohol abuse, anorexia, acne, and more." Though it is not entirely clear from his e-book which he was experiencing during the time of his hospitalization, nor for how long he remained in bed, he writes that a doctor told him, "You will never run further than 100 meters ever again due to your asthma and weak lungs."

He had always been drawn to spiders, mantids, lizards, and other insects. He committed to caring for them because they were so "light and delicate that you could literally kill them just by picking them up wrong." Toward these creatures, he was tender. He had spent enough time analyzing their behavior that he claimed he could "walk up to a jumping spider or a huntsman and tell if it's dehydrated and then present that spider with a teaspoon of water and make it drink. Same with moths and butterflies." I imagine that Harley, as a young child riddled with unnerving symptoms, found comfort in caring for bodies like his, that were mysterious in their fragility. From watching his many interactions with spiders on YouTube over the years, I can envision him crooning *gently, gently, gently, use our hands*, as he encourages a bulbous black spider into his palm, collecting a fragment of web to make him feel at home, and shaping the web into a small circular pallet to make a little bed for him in the middle there.

I can picture this because amid Durianrider's vile and bizarre posts on Instagram—comparing his ex-girlfriend to Amber Heard, fat-shaming Calvin Klein models, or spreading conspiracy theories about COVID-19—he still, in his forties, regularly shares interactions he has with spiders and lizards. He loves Redback spiders, a more toxic Australian variant of Black Widows. He once named a pair of sisters Mary and Sally, and their mum, who had a web nearby, Beth. When their babies emerged he admired them in their multitudes, and when his yard later supported over fifty adult females, he used a spray bottle when the summer heat was at its fiercest to mist them all. A lizard called Bluey eats his fruit scraps, and he once let a spider live in his kitchen for two years, sprinkling the countertops with water so she'd stay hydrated, murmuring, *beautiful little specimen, very friendly little spider as well.*

· * * *

At sixteen, Leanne left her family's farm and moved to Sydney alone. I can imagine that, with the change in geography came an alteration of her internal landscape too, her perception of self affected by the pressures of finding a way to belong in the city, feel desired by men, find out who she truly was on her own. She took a job at McDonald's and ate there twice a day, six days a week for a year, and put on twenty pounds. Her skin broke out in oily bumps. Her body, as she writes in *The Raw Till 4 Diet: Banana Girl Cleanse,* became a "graveyard for innocent tortured animals." As she writes in *My Naked Lunchbox*, she felt lonely during that time, like "a male calf in a veal crate. cold. lost. helpless. starved of proper nourishment, yearning for connection." She took up swimming every morning, which gave her "a euphoric high" and got outside to walk on a regular basis. It was then, during one of her walks, that she noticed "a guy on the path watching the surf." He attempted to talk with her, but Leanne was too shy, and so she kept walking.

The guy was there almost every day, and Leanne got to know him. They started dating. Leanne soon realized he was a drug dealer. She began regularly taking ecstasy, speed, and cocaine. She dropped forty pounds but wanted to lose even more; to her, there was no such thing as too skinny. One day, working her job at the supermarket, she fainted in front of a customer; she had run-walked two and a half hours in the morning and hadn't eaten anything all day. When friends expressed concern, telling Leanne she looked like she would fall down a crack if she kept going, she thought, "Yeh bitches you just jealous," and increased her efforts.

After four or so years of experiencing anorexia, bulimia, and drugs, Leanne broke up with her then-boyfriend. She got breast implants. One night, after her chest had healed, she dressed herself in a "short white crop top with a glitter-filled blue number 1 symbol on it, tight black faux leather pants on the bottom. Fuck-me boots." Her blond hair, now bleached, skimmed her waist. She went out to a nightclub and found herself dancing with a famous Australian cricket player. In *My Naked Lunchbox*, Leanne writes that she "resembled a Barbie doll" and that the attention she received from the player made her feel "worthy, and validated" for a brief moment, before leaving her "empty." "I was now the embodiment of a fuckboi's fantasy," she writes in *My Naked Lunchbox*. "It was bittersweet."

*   *   *

Harley left his childhood home at nearly the same age as Leanne, though his departure was more tumultuous. As he writes in *Carb the Fuck Up*, his teenage years were a blur of drugs and graffiti, paid for in part by designer clothes that he stole and resold. A stint in juvenile prison did nothing to slow his habits, and his mother eventually filed a restraining order against him. Harley moved out suddenly enough at seventeen that he left both his Walkman and bicycle in his mom's house; all he owned were the clothes on his back and the grey and neon yellow Nike Air Max 95s on his feet. Like his beloved spiders, he managed to spin comfort from nearly nothing. That first night alone, he found a spot to bed in the reeds, thinking to himself, "Nature is awesome! It's so fucking cold though."

Not too long after leaving home, a friend offered him shelter in a shed. As Harley fell asleep that night, he remembers thinking about how fortunate he was that his "biggest problem was mosquitoes versus bombs dropping or machete welding [sic] bandits looking for bodies to chop up." He reflects that he "didn't even know what the word gratitude meant back then" but he soon grew familiar with the feeling. "I really started to appreciate things more." He filed for welfare, got a small place of his own, and learned to take care of both himself and his home. He settled down and six months later moved back in with his mother, the time apart and Harley's growth working wonders to mend their relationship.

Without enough money to buy a car or take taxis everywhere he needed to go, Harley dusted off his mountain bike and started cycling around his neighborhood. At eighteen, without any training, the hills initially seemed comparable to Mount Everest, but after a few months of riding, Harley took pride in showing his friends that he could ride up steep inclines with little trouble. Biking expanded his perception of how far he might go—both literally and metaphorically. He began to test his own limits. One day, he set off from his home in O'Halloran Hill, a suburb of Adelaide, and rode south. Accustomed to moving his body to the pulsing bass at raves, I imagine Harley probably felt some thrill in finally making his own rhythm. Rather than feeling buoyed by synthetic highs and the flicker of technicolor lights, his legs throbbed with a new kind of energy. I imagine that the countryside flickered by in a reel of wide swaths of farmland and trees reaching toward the sky.

That day, when Harley reached the town nearest to his, he kept going. After riding nearly fifty kilometers (thirty-one miles), he was overcome with thirst. He had only two dollars with him, which afforded him one sparkling mineral water and a pasty from a gas station. On the way back, he was heartened by a passing group of cyclists on road bikes. Upon taking stock of Harley's tennis shoes, mountain bike, and lack of water, one rider asked, "You local?" The group was impressed he had come so far with so little. Harley kept their encouragement close as he pedaled; he was struggling immensely with fatigue and dehydration. He stopped twenty-seven kilometers from home when he saw an apricot tree by the road and devoured the fruit even though it was half-ripe, each bite crunchy. After falling asleep for a while, he made it back "sun burnt, fatigued, dehydrated, and cranky as hell."

The apricots foreshadowed a life of fruit to come, but Harley wouldn't change his diet just yet. Instead, one year later, in 1997, he smoked some weed. "I instantly regretted it," he writes in *Carb the Fuck Up*. "I missed the sharp feel of clarity from being sober."

*   *   *

In the Garden of Eden, once Eve eats of the fruit at the serpent's suggestion and shares some with Adam, God punishes them for their transgressions. The snake will crawl on his belly for life, the woman will experience painful childbirth, the man will toil at barren ground. Adam and Eve are cast out of the garden with the knowledge that they were and will be dust, with a lifetime of pain and struggle, thorn and thistles to bear in the space between.

After the fall, as Eve's body strained in labor with Cain and then Abel, and as Adam planted seeds just to see them shrivel with poor soil or drought, I wonder if the two of them fought over their choice to bite into wisdom, if they dreamed up scenarios in which they ate from the tree of life instead and became deities or just immortal humans, forever feasting their eyes and tongues on nectar and seed. I can imagine that they longed to get back to the lush land between rivers, limbs heavy with fruit. In the garden, there were no murderous siblings, no floods, no famine, no mysterious illness, no infertility, no bodies that became weak with age. There was no pain.

Who wouldn't yearn to return to such a paradise? To be human is to be persistently aware of the utter vulnerability of a body and to reckon with how privilege and genetics and chance impact the ways in which we move through the world, the rapidity with which we deteriorate. To return to a holy place of wellness would mean being absolved of this knowledge, even if just for a moment. For a person who is wracked with symptoms—say, systemic candida overgrowth, persistent explosive diarrhea, chronic fatigue, and acne—any kind of cure can seem like a mirage in a desert. If you are thirsty enough, sand can take the shape of water and apricots can seem like salvation. A distant promise of relief, even if it's ephemeral, can be enough to keep moving forward one step at a time.

Leanne might have felt this way. At her lowest, rather than being tempted by a snake in a garden, she fell again and again for the ploys of snake-oil salespeople. She tried every diet under the sun: Atkins, Zone Diet, blood-type diet, CSIRO, one that had her eating "livers for breakfast and a whole chicken a day!" She spent "THOUSANDS on natural therapies, Chinese medicine and Ayurvedic Dr's, obese naturopaths, well-meaning homeopaths, and Australia's best Gastroenterologist." Each, which at one point seemed like an oasis in the midst of a vast desert, just left her feeling frustrated and cheated. The men who treated her looked the opposite of healthy. One of her doctors took a smoke break in the middle of her consultation. She purchased $300 worth of supplements from another, and they only clogged up her system. Her gastroenterologist "was fat, looked like an alcoholic and had some obvious skin disorder—all which didn't instill any confidence." He told her she had an inflamed gut and said there was a drug from the United States being released in a few months that might cure her. She told him she had no interest in trying.

Tired of pills, tired of placing all her hope for wellness in men who didn't look as though they cared for their own bodies, and tired of paying vast sums of money for no results, Leanne took matters into her own hands. She quit drugs, alcohol, and coffee. She booked a trip to Greece, where all she wanted was to "finally be healthy and look hot in a bikini." Instead, she ate meat every meal and returned home to Australia "feeling like hell." It was then, in 2006, that she found deliverance. In an alternative magazine, Leanne read an article about a woman who only ate raw food. Leanne believed not only the woman's testimony, but also in her radiance; she looked vibrant on the page.

"I knew in my heart this was it," Leanne writes. "Raw food was going to save the day."

* * *

Imagine just one more origin story. In this beginning, the murmur of rushing water permeates the lush layers of a primordial rainforest. Strangler figs root themselves in bark and rope their way toward the upper levels of the canopy. With heads spiked like small dinosaurs and ochre-colored throats, forest dragons perch on small branches. Umbrella trees' leaves droop toward the ground, and from the bright red pods of a maple silkwood, star-shaped flowers bloom in a constellation. As if by some feat of faith, ferns grow from the surface of large, egg-shaped boulders, their leaves like puckered fabric.

A man makes his way through the jungle. As I envision this scene, slick leaves caress his hips as he wades through ancient flora. Every green plant, every flicker of technicolor feather, every matte scale and gossamer wing and sturdy trunk and glossy shell seek the scarcity of sun that streams through the green above. Each plant here is a testament to time itself; seeds bear witness to prior generations. Between birds chittering, wind rustling leaves, insects chirruping, animals howling, and rain pattering, the space bursts with sound and song. There is a sense of abundance, one the man hasn't encountered in quite this way before. And the man is hungry. He finds a bush turkey nesting with chicks but, outside of observation, finds no desire to consume their flesh. Instead, he forages for low-hanging fruit and tastes an assortment of wild sweetness.

The man is Harley, and Harley has just cycled 2,000 kilometers to reach this place, Mossman Gorge, home to one of the oldest rainforests in the world. The year is 2005. Eight years have passed since he smoked his last joint. During these years, he has proselytized to friends about the benefits of quitting cigarettes, and he has taught them to ride farther and faster. He has biked thousands of kilometers. In the rainforest, he leaves his clothes and bicycle. The moonlit night is humid and warm. Harley is naked and he swims out to a boulder in the middle of the river.

Lying on the rock, he contemplates. *What on earth am I doing? Is a vegan lifestyle some dogma or a pure instinct? Where do I want to be in ten years? How can I help people help themselves more?* In this moment, Harley might not know that his life will be full of cycling and ripe fruits and more followers than he ever might have dreamed of. All he knows is that there is nothing to distract him in this primeval place, no voices other than his own. It is here, on this rock, that he recognizes his life's purpose: "To help people get themselves drug free fit and at the same time we save the animals, society, and the planet."

CHAPTER 10

Banana Island

AFTER FINDING THE ARTICLE ABOUT THE RADIANT RAW FOOD woman, Leanne hungered for more. In 2007, she read books like *Raw Food Detox Diet*, *Sunfood Diet Success System*, and *Raw Energy*. She got on to the internet, where she discovered an Australian raw food forum. She typed so much talking to other members, she says, that her "chubby little fingers were suffering from RSI," a repetitive strain injury. She began making gourmet raw food creations, all of them high in fat, and brought one to a picnic in a park where other raw vegans were meeting up. It was there that she met Nadia, a woman who would later become one of her best friends. Nadia ate ten mangoes at the picnic and nothing else. *What the heck was this chick thinking?* Leanne remembers wondering. Nadia explained that on a high-carb, raw vegan lifestyle, Leanne could eat endless amounts of food; plenitude was the point. But Leanne still had questions. What about all that sugar? Wasn't that bad for her? And what about candida? Diabetes? Her doubts didn't last long. Nadia had an answer for everything, all of it backed up by a book that Leanne would later call her "bible," *The 80/10/10 Diet: Balancing*

Your Health, Your Weight, and Your Life, One Luscious Bite at a Time by Douglas Graham. In it, Graham suggests that people should derive their daily calories from raw food and try to hit daily macronutrient totals of 80% carbohydrates and 10% or less each of protein and fat. In the book, after pages and pages of questions— "Are We Herbivores?" "Are We Starch Eaters?" "Are We Sucklings of Animals?" "Are We Eaters of Nuts, Seeds, and Other High-Fat Plants?"—Graham finally reveals that we are in fact "Frugivores!" Why? Because "humans are sweet seekers by nature." As evidence of this, when Graham offers people tropical fruits, their interest is instant. "Almost invariably," he writes, "I hear something like:

> 'Wow, this is the best thing I have ever tasted!'
> 'I just found my new favorite food!'
> 'I could live on this!'
> 'Where can I get this at home?'
> 'Do you know of any mail-order catalogs that can ship some to me?'
> 'Is this expensive? I want to buy lots of it!'
> 'How do I learn about other fruits like this?'"

If these testimonials aren't enough to demonstrate that humans were created to eat fruit, Graham has a chart to prove it. In a table labeled "Humans vs. Carnivores," Graham reveals that our opposable thumbs "make us extremely well equipped to collect a meal of fruit in a matter of a few seconds," whereas lions cannot. Our colons are "convoluted," while those of carnivores are "smooth." We sleep only eight hours a day, while carnivores "sleep and rest from 18 to 20." In addition to these biological differences, Graham suggests performing an imaginative exercise where you think about a "field of wheat, or a herd of cattle, or a flock of birds in flight." From my interpretation of Graham's book, if you're not salivating over unprocessed golden kernels or the uncooked, feathered wing of a sparrow, it's clear that eating fruit is your destiny.

Though Graham's ideas caught on like wildfire—at least within the high-carb, raw vegan community—they weren't new. In 1880, John Smith published a book, *Substance Of the Work Entitled Fruits And Farinacea, The Proper Food Of Man,* with exactly the same ideas, down to the descriptions of how human teeth compare with those of rats, beavers, and other carnivora. When I asked Graham about the similarities between his book and Smith's in a 2023 interview, he said, "It's not a new idea under the sun."

In the late 1990s and early 2000s, Graham headlined weekend fruitfests, had his own blog, and, in 2006, most famously, published *The 80/10/10 Diet* (commonly referred to by followers as "811"). While the wealth of information he posted online could be a lot for a newcomer to take in, there was a sort of gateway to the lifestyle he created: a trip to Banana Island. It might sound glamorous but, in reality, "a trip to Banana Island" means going to the supermarket to purchase a large quantity of bananas and eating them every morning, afternoon, and night for a week straight. For someone satisfied with their life, their health, and their body, a trip to Banana Island might sound entertaining at best, a wild diet to pitch to the pages of a glossy magazine. But imagine for a moment that you have just survived a litany of trials: messages from the media insisting you must take up less space to be beautiful; a dependence on substances of some kind to get through each day; or a sense of confusion about your purpose in life. Imagine that your body has bloated beyond recognition, erupted in acne, or rebelled in some other way. You visit doctors who do not dig to find the root cause of your symptoms, but instead provide you with medication or speculation. Days blur together in a haze of discomfort. For years, this is what you have endured. You are desperate. You want relief.

Imagine then, that at a picnic, a gorgeous, glowing woman takes the time to listen to your symptoms. It's the first time in too many years to count that someone has been so empathetic. The woman tells you about a plan for wellness you've never heard of before. So later that night, maybe, you Google the diet for yourself, wanting to know more. There are countless blog posts, meetups, and videos in which Douglas Graham and his followers praise the benefits of Banana Island. In one of them, Graham sits beside one of his practitioners, a man in a fitted "LETTUCE TURNIP THE BEET" muscle tank who goes by the name MC Fructose. Behind them are windows that offer a view of a heavily wooded area, the light of day dwindling. Graham's thinning grey hair is pulled back into a ponytail and his white T-shirt looks too big for his frame. On the front, an anthropomorphized pineapple smiles, arms and legs outstretched. The words "RAW PASSION" are spelled out in cartoon bamboo and an array of fruits—mangoes, grapes, oranges, bananas—cascades from the letters.

"People who don't know what Banana Island is, it's a mono-food island. A mono-island is when you eat one food for an extended period of time and Banana Island is with bananas," MC Fructose explains. He turns to Graham. "When do you recommend Banana Island and for who?"

"I use Banana Island as part of—" Graham pauses, purses his mouth, and looks to the ceiling, "an emotional release program that I teach . . . The actual Banana Island program is one where we are looking at the emotional reasons as to why people treat themselves a certain way or why people use food to retreat or to numb themselves or to actually sometimes intentionally hurt themselves. We learn how to separate emotions from memories so we can get free in the moment rather than hanging on to old emotions from the past."

Graham makes clear he doesn't believe Banana Island to be restrictive in any way. People who choose to follow the diet can eat bananas in a variety of different ways—blended, diced, frozen—and they're allowed to eat "some lettuce and celery, maybe some cucumbers." The idea behind Banana Island is that practitioners focus less on food than usual. Because they know what they will be eating, they have more space and time to explore their emotions. Proponents of Banana Island note health benefits, too. A raw vegan named Liz, on her blog *The Raw Herbalist*, writes that Banana Island is intended to "allow our digestive system to have a break. Our digestion typically consumes over 50% of our energy . . . The energy saved by 'going on the island' can be utilized for cleansing the bloodstream, flushing the bowel, detoxing, reducing water retention and healing the gut, which is the root cause of most diseases."

Taking a trip to the island, according to Graham, can help people learn how much fruit is necessary for them to feel full, get used to eating only raw food, and learn how to cycle through ripened food. In his interview with MC Fructose, Graham explains, "People can do it on their own pretty safely for a week. They might do two weeks."

Leanne, after attending the picnic, ate only bananas for almost a month.

*   *   *

In my desperation—and, I would guess, in Leanne's—Banana Island looked more inviting than the slew of pills offered to me by doctors. Even though I hadn't met him, Douglas Graham (or Dr. D, as he called himself) seemed like he really cared about the people who joined him in paradise. Much of Leanne and Harley's views on health were shaped by Graham's teachings, so as I visited the 30BaD website, the concept of 811 became familiar enough that it started to make a kind of sense. Maybe I *could* purify my body if only I ate a little better. Even if I didn't go all in on Banana Island, maybe reducing fats in my diet could help my body cure itself or lessen the load of digestion so that my brain could have the time, space, and resources to heal. It seems silly to write now (of course eating only bananas wouldn't miraculously heal me), but the way Graham—and subsequently Leanne—talked about potential cures was nothing new. Instead, their hope for healing grew from the same soil that gave Cornelius Valkenburg de Villiers Dreyer the confidence to believe fervently in fruit, or Benedict Lust the desire to offer a menagerie of "purifying" treatments to the public. And I mean this literally. Graham's 811 diet, as well as his philosophy on how to treat illness, came straight from the same source that had Johanna Brandt sailing to the United States to preach the power of grapes: naturopathy.

The story goes like this: Halfway around the world from Leanne and Harley, in 1990, vegan author Victoria Moran boarded a Greyhound bus headed for Marathon, Florida, a city in the Keys. Unlike many tourists, the goal of her trip wasn't to witness the Loggerhead turtles nesting on the beach or to savor a piece of key lime pie after a meal of freshly caught crabs. Instead, she was traveling in pursuit of healthfulness; she wanted to release herself from impurities like "smog and smokers, smorgasbords and self-doubt." At the bus stop, awaiting her arrival, was none other than Douglas Graham—on a tandem bike. After overcoming her initial surprise at his mode of transportation, Victoria's suitcase was tied with an inner tube to the bike, so she straddled the empty seat, and realized "there was only one thing to do—pedal like the dickens."

The pair cycled down Aviation Boulevard, turned onto a road aptly named Mango Lane, and then took a right onto Bruce Drive. At last, they arrived at an oasis of sorts, a two-story house called Club Hygiene, which functioned both as Graham's primary residence and as a health center. The downstairs included a small recreation room, a porch for dining, one bathroom, and three bedrooms featuring two beds each, making it so that six guests could stay at a time. Graham lived upstairs with a rotating crew of three "interns" who helped clean the house, prepare food, and sometimes sought treatments of their own. Guests had access to everything but an oven. There was "a ski machine, a trampoline . . .bikes, boats, decks

a public health figure. He was part of the temperance movement, which scorned partaking in alcohol as sinful, but he soon started to think that eating meat was just as bad; it was a sign of gluttony. He preached that people should, like Adam and Eve, eat only plants, that they should abstain from "exciting" activities like sex or masturbation, and that they should bathe often, get regular doses of sunlight, have access to fresh air, read "non-arousing" books and, as his name might give away, eat graham crackers. While all of this seems like relatively fine advice, Sylvester's delivery of this information was apparently a different story. "He had an excessive vanity," Mildred V. Naylor writes in an article published in 1942. "He considered anyone who did not agree with him an enemy who was determined to cheat him of the glory that was rightfully his." Once, when Sylvester was lecturing in Boston, a group of people came to ridicule him. His followers, Grahamites, so fervent in their belief of both his moral teachings and him as their leader, poured slaked lime out the windows onto the growing mob, which could cause chemical burns. While Sylvester was crusading for moral and bodily salvation, a man named William Alcott was publishing prolifically about the importance of eating only vegetables and drinking only water. Alcott and Sylvester, from the 1830s to 1850s, served as ambassadors of hygienic living.

Flashy mass-produced food and sanitariums aside, at their core, hygienics believed in preventative care through "vegetarianism, sunlight, frequent bathing, regular exercise, fresh air, dress reform, and sex health." Practitioners of natural hygiene believe that our bodies, particularly our organs, are always working to cleanse toxins from our systems, but that if too many toxins build up, we experience "acute disease" like "cancer and emphysema." This can only be fought by "life energy," which young people have in abundance. Young people "have rapid, dramatic 'healing crises,' such as vomiting or 24-hour colds" that hygienics view as evidence of self-healing. Older people "perform this cleansing less effectively and can develop chronic ailments like asthma, arthritis, adult-onset diabetes and digestive disorders." In the worldview of hygienics, the only way to stave off disease and regain life energy is to eat mostly raw food, sunbathe, and exercise.

In the late 1800s and early 1900s, the different sects of naturopathy weakened in strength when each of their founders died, and the rise in public awareness of scientific concepts like germ theory meant that people had more information on which to base their own personal health decisions. However, natural hygiene was reintroduced to a mainstream audience in the 1980s by Harvey and Marilyn Diamond, then husband and wife, who wrote the nutrition book *Fit for Life* in which they advocated that people should eat mostly raw fruit, avoid combining proteins and carbohydrates, and avoid dairy. Graham's food philosophy at Club Hygiene (the name itself a nod to the health beliefs he subscribed to) was largely similar; guests in reasonably good health who stayed at the center ate mostly raw fruit, extraordinarily large salads, and a few nuts every day, while those deemed to be in poor health were told to sunbathe and fast. During her stay, Moran was treated to a veritable buffet of fresh, cleansing foods. She ate red and white cabbage slaw dressed in a light cashew dressing; smoothies made from frozen mangoes and bananas, blended up with water; fruit from the garden; and watermelon.

After meals, there was no need to wash plates or utensils with soap, because they "didn't need it with raw foods." The time saved from not having to cook or clean was spent in more nourishing ways. Moran tried keeping up with Graham for seventeen miles on a bike, gales of wind against the pair for much of the distance. Alert and inspired from the food and exercise, she "eagerly borrowed Graham's computer for 'creative, useful work.'" At night, with the other guests, Moran played Pictionary, listened to classical music, watched *Betty Boop,* or took "walks timed to catch the awesome island sunset or to smell the night-blooming jasmine."

After spending two weeks with Graham at the center, Moran

returned to the bus stop, her suitcase full of papaya and ripe red bananas. She was convinced that following a hygienic lifestyle was a form
of self-love and felt "lean and strong, rested and healthy."

Not everyone who visited was so lucky.

*   *   *

In 1993, within the Division of Administrative Hearings, Douglas N.
Graham is listed as the Respondent in a "matter" that "came before
the Board of Chiropractic . . .on December 10, 1998, in Naples,
Florida." The case details the treatment of two people referred to as
"patients" by the court documents (though, in a 2023 Zoom interview,
Graham said, "These people were not patients"). The first is a twenty-
five-year-old woman identified as K.E. in court documents, who
arrived at the health center on December 7, 1992. Court documents
state that K.E. was a walk-in patient who, "due to a lack of funds . . .
declined further chiropractic care." Though K.E. was suffering from
myriad symptoms, including "occasional dizziness and headache;
occasional pain between shoulders; frequent constipation and
difficult digestion, with occasional pain over stomach; occasional
colds, ear noises, and sore throat; occasional skin eruptions (rash);
occasional frequent urination; and occasional cramps or backache
and vaginal discharge, with frequent irregular menstrual cycle," but
K.E. really only wanted help with one thing: her back. "They said
I had scoliosis when I was young," she remembers telling Graham.
"I'm curious if it still is there."

Court documents state that the appointment lasted around
twenty minutes. Graham checked her spine and talked to her about
her diet, but did not record his observations, a diagnosis, or a plan
of treatment. Instead, either that day or soon after, he offered K.E. a
six-month internship with him. In exchange for his nutritional and
medical advice, she would live on the second floor of Club Hygiene,

make the guests' beds, clean the bathrooms, help prepare food, and check the guests' blood pressure daily. During the internship, her symptoms persisted. She had difficulty digesting and was often constipated. She turned to Graham and his assistant, an unlicensed naturopath who called himself Dr. Tim Trader, for advice. In a 2023 interview, I asked Graham if he knew Trader was an unlicensed naturopath and he responded, "Yeah, I knew a fair bit about Tim." They told her she would be cured through raw food, but her new diet brought no relief. Over the course of three months, her weight dropped to 92 pounds.

If you are sick enough, Natural Hygienists believe that fasting is the only way to rid your body of toxins. During a fast, a "patient" is only allowed to drink water. In April 1993, four months after starting her internship, K.E. was advised to stop eating. Graham, who admitted that "he had not done any examination that would permit him to appropriately treat K.E.," told her she "had severe problems, including but not limited to, malabsorption syndrome, leaky gut syndrome, potential hiatal hernia, and resultant malnutrition," though these findings or reasoning for treatment were not recorded anywhere. During the hearing, Graham insisted that K.E. had been "his maid" the entire time, and therefore he shouldn't be held to any sort of standard of medical practice. In a 2023 interview, when I asked Graham if K.E. had been a patient, he said no. He told me that K.E. had been a friend of Tim Trader's and that "she thought that some kind of relationship was going to happen that never did. She got very upset and so she turned her vengeance on me."

K.E.'s weight dropped to a dangerously low 87 pounds due to her two-week fast, and it continued to plummet even after she began to eat again. She grew concerned and, according to court documents, "sought to consult with Frank Sabatino, D.C., another 'hygienic physician' . . .and also a medical doctor; however their findings are not of record." Evidence of the impact of the fast or any "subsequent care" required by K.E. as a result was not introduced to the Board, but an onlooker noted that her physical presence at the hearing "evidenced good health." She left Club Hygiene soon after and filed a legal complaint in 1996.

When I interviewed Graham in 2023, he claimed that "eventually, under oath," K.E. said "none of this ever happened, none of the allegations that I put forth were ever, you know, they weren't real. I'm backing out of this entire thing." When I asked Graham if he had those documents in his possession, his response was, "No."

* * *

Graham, in his own life, found raw food and subsequently the principles of Natural Hygienics. In a 2023 interview, he described dabbling in vegetarianism and a vegan diet, including cooked food, before he realized that raw was the way. He used a metaphor of two tuning knobs on a radio; when he gave up pasta and potatoes, and swapped cooked food for raw, he dialed in. "Everything just fell into place," he told me. His coordination, memory, and physical skills improved, and his need for sleep became less. He felt so incredible, so excited about these changes, that he wanted everyone else to feel similarly. During his chiropractic training, while talking with a friend over lunch one day, he shared his philosophy that if people were put on an island and "just ate fruits and vegetables and they were physically active and got some sleep . . .they'd get healthy as all heck." The friend gave him a name for what he was describing: Natural Hygiene. To Graham, "Hygiene always meant the science of human health . . .Hygiene is always, make intelligent choices."

Club Hygiene was born from Graham's desire to create an island, a haven, where people could practice these principles. Court documents describe Club Hygiene as a place where a "hygienic (nutritionally

sound) lifestyle based on the consumption of uncooked fruit and vegetables, nuts and seeds" was promoted as well as "fasting (to detoxify
the body)." To support his methods, Graham earned his Doctor of
Chiropractic from Life Chiropractic College in Marietta, Georgia,
and in an interview with me, shared that he "studied fasting in the
medical program" and was "licensed to conduct fasts in the state of
Florida." He also shared that he has a "Doctorate in Health" from the
University of Natural Health, a program, according to him, "based on
old-time Hygiene." The present-day University of Natural Health website does not list "Doctorate in Health" as a degree option, and when I
reached out to Graham to clarify the specific title, he responded, "The
degree was bestowed a long time ago." While by Graham's admission
and as evidenced by the court documents he had all the requisite training and licensure for his two chiropractic practices, he emphasized
that a person referred to in court documents as B.D. (Brian) was not a
patient. "They never came to my office," he told me. "They never saw
me professionally."

Instead, Graham claims that Brian had "stayed . . .at Club
Hygiene for a little while" six years prior. At that time, Graham
provided "nutritional consulting and lifestyle monitoring" and in a
subsequent second visit, the two "made closer friends." In his third
and final visit, Graham claims that Brian called him and said, "Can
I come visit you, I'm kind of in a bad way." Graham explained to
me that Brian had just spent a month in the hospital, and that his
medical records at the time were "two words from a medical doctor
on a sheet of paper that said, 'Good luck.'" According to the court
documents, Brian arrived at Club Hygiene on November 7, 1993,
almost exactly one year after K.E. Thirty-seven years old, 5'9½" tall,
and only 115 pounds, Brian "was in extremely poor health." The
court documents state that Brian was HIV positive and had developed AIDS, but Graham testified "he was unaware." When I asked

Graham in 2023 if he knew Brian was HIV positive, he responded, "We did not discuss HIV six years prior." Court documents note that Graham's testimony about this matter was "rejected as inherently improbable and unworthy of belief."

Though Graham claims Brian was not being treated as a patient, court records show that Brian communicated an "anal infection, frequent diarrhea, weight loss, inability to assimilate food, fatigue, and loss of energy" as symptoms and that an examination "confirmed the presence of an anal infection (thought to be fungal in origin) oozing clear fluid and further noted . . .an irritated nose and throat (slight redness) and that the upper cervical and lower lumbar were tender and fixated." In his "only recommendation reflected by the patient records," Graham suggested "daily light massage, muscle release, and gentle specific adjustments." Court records make it clear that Brian began fasting, but when I asked Graham if he suggested the fast, he said "No. I can't tell you where that idea came from. The idea of doing those things is an old idea. When you don't feel well, a lot of times you skip meals or just want something to drink."

B.D. drank only water for nine days, according to court records, and withered to 102.5 pounds. He drank "diluted apple and celery juice" to break his fast, and continued drinking juice for seven days, during which time he lost another two and a half pounds. When I asked Graham why Brian's weight and blood pressure were recorded if Brian was not his patient, Graham responded, "He weighed himself." When I followed up by remarking that I might not take a friend's weight and blood pressure daily in my home and record it, Graham responded, "No, but you're not a doctor, so of course you wouldn't." When I responded affirming that he was a doctor, Graham responded, "I am a doctor, but that doesn't make everybody my patient."

On November 23, Brian began eating solid food. From then to December 6, Brian's blood pressure dropped lower and lower. He slept most days and started to have a difficult time breathing. Patient notes from November 30 indicate all four quadrants of Brian's lungs had blockages as a result of mucus or foreign bodies, what could indicate a clear sign of pneumonia. Graham "suggested he go to a hospital," but Brian said he didn't want to. Even when Brian's fingertips started turning blue, Graham did not call for any additional help. "We just kind of watched him," Graham said in court. "There was not a lot any of us could do at this point."

Court records state that on December 6, 1993, "B.D.'s blood pressure is noted as 62/52 and pulse/respiration as 100/weak. B.D. is again noted as very fatigued, and his weight is recorded as 95 ¼ pounds." Graham disputes this timeline. When I asked him in 2023 about Brian's last visit to Club Hygiene, he said, "Within hours of his coming, maybe a day or two of his coming to visit, he was really not well . . . and I did the appropriate thing which was to send him to the hospital." When I followed up by referring to the court records that indicate Brian stayed at Club Hygiene for a month, Graham responded, "No." When I asked why no one had called the hospital if Brian had been at Club Hygiene for one month, Graham responded, "He had just come from a month in the hospital. I told you up front . . . He certainly didn't want to go until I said, 'Brian, you've gotta go. You've gotta go, man. I mean there's no Hail Mary here.'"

On December 7, 1993, someone called an ambulance, though Graham, when asked in the hearing who, said, "I have no idea." When I spoke with Graham in 2023, he confirmed this, saying, "There were five or six people working in Club Hygiene at the time. I'm not sure who called." EMTs noted "breathing diff[iculty]" and Brian was taken directly to the emergency room. He remained at Fishermen's Hospital for thirteen days, during which time his condition showed no signs of improving. His discharge summary describes him as an "emaciated 37-year-old male who is on a non rebreather oxygen mask." With fluid in his lungs, "confused regarding his recent medical history," Brian's prognosis was poor. He was "admitted to Lower Florida Keys Health System, Key West, Florida, at 2:50 p.m., December 20, 1993. Thereafter, his condition deteriorated, and at 9:17 p.m., December 26, 1993, he was pronounced dead."

*   *   *

Graham's license to practice as a chiropractor was suspended for one year, followed by two years of probation. He was fined one thousand dollars. In our 2023 conversation, Graham stated that after the verdict, he went to the Florida Chiropractic Board and claims they ended up ruling that he could continue his practice and have his "paperwork monitored for six months." In those years, Graham was lecturing almost full time, so chose instead to sell his practice. "I don't really need anyone monitoring my paperwork," he told me, "but neither of these people were patients to begin with."

He opened a new retreat center in Costa Rica. In 2011, on an online message board, someone with the username Steve asked about a "recent death @ Dougs fasting retreat?" (indicating Doug Graham's fasting retreat) where a participant passed away after "an episode of some sort" during a walking tour following a fast. Graham responded, "When someone dies on a bus, has a heart attack or whatever, is it the driver's fault? If they die in a movie theater, is the cinema at fault? A woman attended my fasting event. She got better, as expected, and wrote a glowing report. She decided to stay for my Walking Tour event. During that event, she had an episode of some type." When I asked Graham about this post during our 2023 interview, he confirmed the report. "Yes, she had a heart problem and died in the hospital," he told me. He described her as a medical doctor who attended the walking tour with her partner. "Her partner told me that she specifically told no one, including me, about her heart problem from twenty years prior because she didn't want to give it the energy that it could gain by her talking about it. She didn't want to claim it, she didn't want to own it, didn't want to talk about it."

During our interview, I asked Graham if the situations involving K.E., Brian, or the Walking Tour attendee had prompted him to think about the responsibility that he holds or if it encouraged him to take medical reports before people attended his events in order to safeguard himself against claims made against him. He responded, "No. Do we learn from experience? Yes, I hope I learn from every experience. Do I want to stop trusting people because somebody burned me? No, I don't stop trusting . . . Do I act as responsibly as possible when providing services to people? Most certainly. But I'm not in private practice at the moment . . . I'm not functioning as a doctor. I am a doctor. I have those qualifications, I have that knowledge, but that doesn't make everybody I meet my client or my patient or my anything."

When I asked whether or not he considers the people who attend his fasting retreats his patients, he responded, "I wouldn't even begin to call them my patients."

When I asked what people paying to attend his retreats are expecting if not medical care, he responded, "They are expecting somebody who has been up that mountain to consult with them and guide them through a positive experience."

Following my Zoom conversation with Graham, I emailed him to ask why, given that he emphasized that fasting participants were "not patients," and that he does not "charge for medical services or provide such care," or is "not practicing" medicine, why he felt it important to still go by Dr. Doug Graham. I also asked whether or not he thought, if by using the title of "Dr.," he was leading people to believe they were receiving medical care when, in some contexts, he is adamant that they aren't. He responded, "When I graduated from Life Chiropractic College, now Life University, the exact words at graduation were, 'Students, rise.' Then we took a vow. We were then told, 'Doctors, you may sit down.' Doctor became part of my name. Something like being knighted by the queen, when you become a Sir, and the title becomes part of your name. No, I am not misleading anyone, and I make my position perfectly clear."

*   *   *

In January 2014, after paying the $8,000 entry fee, Leah Hodge traveled from Australia to Costa Rica to participate in a fast supervised by Graham and the Walking Tour that followed. She had attended Graham's talk at the Woodstock Fruit Festival in 2013 and was convinced that he could help her heal from ulcerative colitis. "I needed to do this to heal myself and live a proper life," she shared in a YouTube video made after the event. She disclosed her health condition on the application form and claims that five minutes after sending in her information she received an acceptance email. (When I asked Graham if he takes health histories before people fast, he said yes, and when I asked if he ever denies anyone from fasting, he said, "Sure. Fasting is inappropriate for a phenomenal number of people, for a huge number of reasons.") During her twenty-five-day fast, Hodge claims she experienced daily bouts of bloody diarrhea and nausea that left her weak and exhausted, as she was unable to sleep. When I asked Graham what he remembered about her fast, he said it was "relatively rough." When I asked if a "relatively rough" fast was normal, he said, "Most fasts are uneventful. But almost all fasts have some rough moments or rough days. So, is it normal? Yeah, it's normal to have a rough fast . . .but she came out of it pretty well."

Breaking the fast seemed a light at the end of a tunnel for Hodge. She cried with relief when she was told she could eat. (Graham emphasizes that it is each individual's choice to fast. "I don't enforce fasting on anyone," he told me. "Never have and never will.") The introduction of food brought even more pain for Hodge. She couldn't keep anything down. "I remember feeling so alone and helpless and like I was going to die," Hodge said in a YouTube video. "I had no energy left." Other fasters who had started eating again were able to lift weights and run, but Hodge claims she couldn't walk farther than two steps without fainting. Hodge claims that Graham did not personally come to check on her, but instead sent his interns, who Hodge says were emotionally helpful, but had no medical knowledge. Graham, in our 2023 interview, denied this claim. When I read him Hodge's allegations and asked if he checked on her, he responded, "We check on every faster three times per day." I asked if he personally checked on her or if an intern did, and he said, "Both." When I asked if his interns had medical training or were trained to respond to people who were fasting, Graham responded, "I've had interns who are doctors. I've had interns who were nurses. I've had interns who were just people off the street. It's not a requirement to have medical training. Why?"

Hodge, in her YouTube video, claims that she was instructed to drink celery and romaine juice; she threw it up. Her mother flew from Australia to Costa Rica to check on her, and was alarmed to see her daughter pale, weak, and unable to walk. Graham confirmed this detail. "As is common when outsiders see people who have fasted, they kind of freak because people who are normally 120 pounds are down to 90 or people who are normally 180 are down to 120. It looks bad," Graham said. "Her mom came and her mom kind of freaked. Her mom was a nurse, felt that she knew a lot of medical stuff, and said, 'Oh, we've got to get you to the hospital.' I said, 'I'm not recommending the hospital because Leah's doing okay, it's just early days of breaking a fast. But if you want to go to a hospital, certainly, by all means, go to a hospital.'"

The pair got into a taxi and traveled five hours to a hospital. Hodge claims Graham told her to lie about fasting, but he firmly denies this claim. "I told her . . . that she was going to respond rather strongly to any medications she might have and she might want to tell them that she tends to hyper react, she tends to react strongly and could they start with perhaps a child's dose," he told me in a 2023 interview. Hodge claims that one doctor found her case too overwhelming, so he passed her along to a second doctor who, upon seeing the color of her skin, recognized that she had a serious infection. Blood test results came back confirming his diagnosis. He urged her to get on antibiotics, but Hodge was so immersed in what she had taken away from Graham's teachings that she worried they were bad for her body. Dehydrated, experiencing acute renal failure and septicimia, Hodge stayed in the hospital for days and later went to the hospital again in Australia to follow up. When she asked Graham for a refund, she claims he denied her unless she signed an NDA. When I asked Graham about this, he responded, "Those are two unrelated things."

More interesting than studying these situations in isolation is thinking about the greater systems that surround and inform them. In the U.S., issues like the high cost of treatment, insurance policies tied to employment, structural racism that has a direct effect on access and quality of healthcare, and more, impact how probable it is that a person might receive timely and meaningful engagement with a doctor or trained medical professional. These factors are compounded by the proliferation of fear-mongering social media posts from people who, though they might have platforms, often have no credible training or education related to the advice they dispense. Vulnerable populations whose views on medical institutions have been shaped in myriad ways might be tempted, as I was, to blame their own bodies for illness and try treatments like fasting, extreme diet changes, juicing, etc. in an attempt to find relief.

The issue, in part, is that these alternative treatment methods—though they certainly can provide different forms of healing, depending on the context—are largely unregulated. In my view, this raises ethical questions. What is the line between personal responsibility for patients and that of someone professing to know of a treatment regimen that might offer a person relief from a specific set of symptoms? What role do individuals have in doing their own research on medical practitioners before partaking in treatment? How are those of us seeking healing supposed to be able to tell a potentially harmful form of intervention from a valuable source of relief, especially when language customarily associated with medical institutions is employed without the support of traditional forms of education or training? Where do the positive benefits of believing in a potential cure end and the real threat of harm begin? Whose responsibility is it to care for patients who have been turned away for lack of insurance, or who are thousands of dollars in debt to a medical system they believe did nothing for them? Who will listen to patients who have been dismissed, ignored, and left to deal with life-altering symptoms on their own? In light of a healthcare system that has failed so many, are alternative cures, untested or untrue, a form of predation? Or is even the promise of relief, the flitting moments of tenderness someone might be shown in the process worth it if the experience brings someone the slightest amount of comfort?

*   *   *

Leanne first encountered Graham and his 811 teachings on a raw food forum. She was intrigued not only by the sheer quantity of fruit he ate ("something like 10 bananas, 10 mangoes, etc.") but also because "a guy on there was insulting him . . .Little did he know that he was doing some great advertising for Dr. D. and the 811 lifestyle!" At the time, for them and many others, Graham's teachings were life-giving. Once on Banana Island, Leanne began to see results. She felt "fit, healthy and well just plain awesome!" The ebb of her symptoms was enough to keep her on a high-fruit lifestyle for nine months, but she soon grew frustrated that she wasn't losing weight. So instead of eating copious amounts of fruit like she was supposed to, she fell back into old habits and began to restrict. The restricting led to cravings and the cravings led to binges. One night, for example, she visited two different sushi places so she could eat thirty veggie plates; she was embarrassed to eat them all in one sitting. With the bingeing came purging, and Leanne felt like she had returned to a particular kind of hell. "To be frank," she writes, "it was fucking soul destroying."

A Tony Robbins seminar saved her. Robbins taught Leanne to manifest her dreams and attract abundance. For thirty days after, she exclusively ate mango and watermelon. She began to reconsider her relationship with Harley, who was then just a friend she had met on a raw food forum. They went out to an open-air market together, where durian was arranged in neat rows. In the video of this date, the dynamics of filming foreshadow years and years of what's to come: Harley is behind the camera and Leanne is his subject. He decides what to hold in frame: flesh of fruit, contours of Leanne's body. This footage, unlike what will come, is not performative. Leanne is not dancing in front of the camera in a bikini or draped across the floor, the camera zooming in on her lean abdomen. Instead, she is wearing a green tank top, black bra straps peeking out. Her face is flushed with what looks like health: Her cheeks hold color, and her smile comes easily. She seems eager for Harley to sit down, to cut into the pungent pods placed before him.

After spending more and more time together, Harley told Leanne, "I really like you." When he said those words, something clicked for Leanne. "I realized I liked him in the same way," she writes. (Harley tells this story crudely. In a video posted years after their first date, he explains, "I remember when I first met Freelee, before I'd go and hang out with her, I used to fap off, clear the pipes, pop the banana, empty out some coconut cream. That is a good tip, guys . . . then you'll know if you're hanging out with them for sexual reasons or just because you find them cool.") Evidently, they found each other cool. They started dating.

Leanne and Harley renamed themselves Freelee The Banana Girl and Durianrider. They began to vlog. In her first YouTube video, Freelee sits in front of a window darkened by night. The camera is close enough that only her face and the tops of her shoulders are in frame.

"Hi, my name is Freelee," she says, introducing herself with the name that will be associated with her public persona. She seems shy; she casts her eyes downward as she speaks. "I'd like to talk to you about why I eat a low-fat raw vegan diet." A chorus of frogs begin singing in the background, threatening to overpower her voice. Rather than meet them with any animosity, Freelee smiles. "It's a pretty cool backdrop, actually," she says, and joins the choir.

CHAPTER 11

The Fruititionist

WHEN I INITIALLY SHOWED 30BAD TO ANDREA, IT LANDED JUST the way I had hoped. We both were delighted by Freelee's offer of two thirty-minute Skype calls and access to her private "fruititionist" website for only $650 per month, along with the general quirkiness of the site—Freelee and Durianrider caricatured (a cartoon Freelee is wearing a skimpy strapless bikini top labeled "vegan," featuring ample cleavage, bombshell blond hair, and a six-pack), the "steam room" where forum members were allowed to swear (elsewhere they were told to use grawlixes like "@#$%^&"), or Freelee's book cover featuring her wearing a strapless dress with the pattern of a watermelon. We wondered about the logistics of navigating life as a fruit-eater. In her videos, Freelee was always conveniently in her kitchen or on her couch, able to spend ample time chugging an entire blender full of bananas or "dateorade," but were normal people like us supposed to cart thirty bananas to class as a casual lunch? What about groceries? How were you supposed to buy enough fruit to last the week and make sure you ate it before it went bad? We spent several dinners together teasing out the details, laughing about the different forums we found (like

"How often should I eliminate?" in which followers posted things like, "I'm eliminating right now!!" or "I only go about twice a day right now. Looking forward to more."). We co-opted phrases like "go fruit yourself" for use in our own life. In these ways, 30BaD offered me a form of connection—if not with other fruit bats on the internet, with Andrea.

Outwardly, the website remained a joke. But when Andrea was at school, I got sucked in. In those moments, the reality of my situation pressed on me more than other times. My vision was clouded by an immediate sense of want. I wanted to get up out of my chair. I wanted to get back to a full course load at school. I wanted to resolve my symptoms. On especially sunny days, I wished I could leave the carpeted hush of my room and go for a run; I hadn't visited the farmlands since marathon training the semester before. Running had been a form of rebellion against my illness, a way of articulating anger. Now I felt deflated somehow, resigned to rest until I received more answers about what was going on. I was sick enough that I knew leaving the apartment would only mean someone would have to pick me up; I wouldn't risk that. At the time I found Freelee and Durianrider, I held myself in the lowest esteem. As an athlete, I felt like I had "given up" and not pushed through to victory. As a woman who had just entered her twenties, I had only kissed a handful of guys freshman year and had remained celibate—first by choice, and then by circumstance. I didn't know how to see myself as worthy of being loved when I didn't have any proof of why I was good. All my former markers of worth like grades and mile splits or the physical ability to do favors for friends rather than frequently being on the receiving end had dissipated. I was left with just me. Me, in a wheelchair.

From a place of twisted curiosity, I followed links from the 30BaD page to Durianrider and Freelee's separate blogs, YouTube channels, and social media pages. Every day, I let myself search each site in my browser and lean back for a tilt-a-whirl of fruit-forward, anti-fat content.

I started with Durianrider, whose public persona intimidated me just as much as it intrigued me. While on some level I found his posts offensive or off-putting, another part of me was lured in by the rhythm of his speech and the sureness he held in his beliefs, especially in his earliest YouTube videos. His first, aptly titled, "Durianrider First Ever YouTube Video June 23rd 2008 #retro," starts off with grainy footage of a spiral-cut pineapple on a stick. "Juicy pineapple in Thailand," Durianrider says to the camera's microphone. "I got the only one with no plastic." He turns the lens to his face, which gives the impression that he's talking just to you, a friend. His face is clear of blemishes and the tip of his nose and cheekbones are lightly bronzed by sun. His eyes are a deep blue. "Let's go check out a fruit market," he says, before the eight seconds of footage cuts out.

The second video he ever posted—this one nineteen seconds long—starts with more grainy footage of fruit: dragonfruit glowing pink; heaps of dark purple, perfectly spherical mangosteen; clusters of khaki-colored longan; piles of limes; and more. "Are you gonna eat this?" Durianrider asks us about the fruit before panning his camera until he lands on strips of raw meat laid out on a metal table. "Or this?" He shows us a Tupperware full of raw meat, a bowl of meat-covered bones, and then two plastic bags of blood, puffed up with air like a bag of goldfish won at a fair. Watching, I remember feeling a sense of calm wash over me. He had distilled the world into right and wrong—evil meat or holy fruit. While the murkiness of my own health left me feeling like I was fumbling in the dark for an answer, this choice seemed simple. "Bag of blood there," Durianrider says in the video. "I don't know about that. Pineapple looks good to me."

Other early video titles of Durianrider's include:

why they call me durianrider
DURIANRIDER STEALS DURIANS
primal diet is for freaks

Raw food lifestyle 101: Durian dinner by candlelight
durianrider: is raw food diet sustainable?

In them, he films himself yet again at the market, challenging anyone on a "primal diet" to come eat from a pile of flesh. He zooms in to show the texture of bone; the roughness of what looks to be tongue; a vibrant, slick, maroon organ; and mounds of pink-and-red-striated meat. "Yeah, get it in ya," Durianrider urges in his Australian accent. He laughs. "That's sick, man. Meat is murder, man. Keep it raw." In a different clip, he explains his moniker by filming himself cycling with a cart of durian strapped to the back of his bicycle. In another, with a yellow and green Specialized helmet strapped to his head, yellow cycling glasses on his forehead, he starts a rhythmic bit of dialogue, saying, "Raw vegan, that's what I am. Mother Nature never broke the heart that loved her. I'm vegan not 'cause some book said it's healthy or whatever. I'm vegan because my heart says it's the right thing to do. So I do it no matter what anyone else says." To those who are meat eaters, he says he can send them an organic meal that very day. The camera swings to show a dead possum on the side of the road, mouth open and organs bursting through its midsection. "It's even got some probiotic culture in there or something," Durianrider jokes.

His personal blog, DURIANRIDER'S BLOG, which he created in 2008, featured his YouTube videos as well as other links. By early 2012, the blog had 235,333 hits and featured the tagline, "Not even 2 lawsuits have shut this blog down..the TRUTH must go on.." A faded grey background marked by white scratches, black font, and red accents gave the site a feeling of intensity, and I remember feeling skeptical or wary of the tone, as it felt combative. His posts ranged from pointed celebrations of personal athletic accomplishments (like "Durianrider wins gruelling 34KM mountain running race," which was then tagged "low carb," "paleo diet," and "primal blueprint" as a means of enticing followers of those diets to see he had won on "Dates and water" alone) to posts riddled with anti-fat rhetoric, like "Fat you eat is the fat you wear . . . effortlessly" or "Eating too much fruit makes you fat! A big fat fatso. Like Freelee." The part of me that had not yet started to unravel my own tangled relationship between thinness, health, and athleticism was compelled to click on the links he posted.

If I conjure them up now, the websites I was browsing exist as a montage of '90s design: blue hyperlinked material, Times New Roman font, bright-colored graphics in neon green or orange that don't fit the rest of the site's aesthetic, and banner ads at the top of the page. There were ads for seminars, summits, meet-ups, DVDs, and online courses. There were graphics featuring "before and after" images, "AS SEEN ON CNN," and testimonials from clients. Authors of each site asked questions like, "Is X really healthy?" or featured pseudoscientific explanations for different digestion processes. There were sites where medical doctors used their credibility to tout nutrition plans that were unrelated to their areas of specialty. There was language about stopping certain kinds of disease, freeing your arteries, and feeling leaner, healthier, and living longer. At the time, rather than being able to see through the gimmicks or pseudoscience, the language on the websites seemed to blend with my own ways of perceiving my body. I viewed something within myself as "bad" or "wrong"; there simply could be no other explanation for why I was so sick, and without reasonable cause.

I became fixated on oil. I began to vilify all forms of it, and considered it a toxin that would clog my arteries and my digestion. In a warped and misinformed echo of the messages about digestion I had received from the doctor in Peru, I began to wonder if oil was somehow slowing the movement of blood to my brain. Looking back, these anxieties are far-fetched, but they were easier to grapple with than the state of my health as a whole or the way that past traumas had bled into my present reality.

While I didn't express my demonization of food to anyone or seek legitimate nutritional help at the time, while writing this book, I sought insight from James and Dahlia Marin, co-founders of the plant-based integrative practice Married to Health. James Marin, COO, is a registered dietitian and environmental nutritionist and Dahlia Marin, CEO, is a registered dietitian nutritionist (RDN). I talked with them about the ways that language can shape our relationship to food—in positive and negative ways. Dahlia, who has been an RDN for over ten years, has worked with thousands of patients, many of whom enter her practice by saying something like, "I've heard X is bad."

"It's a very absolute statement," Dahlia told me over Zoom. "Naming foods 'good' and 'bad' really attaches a lot of emotion to that food, where then someone will say, 'Oh, I've been bad.' They feel like they are bad because they've eaten 'bad' food." To avoid a cycle of shame, Dahlia recommends people speak about food with more objective language, like "inflammatory," so that the choice does not reflect your character but instead describes a reaction that your body might have.

Dahlia also talked about the importance of evaluating health claims made by people who tout their credentials online. "Just because somebody promoting something is a healthcare provider doesn't mean that it is completely evidence-based," she explained. "Does this person have a well-rounded picture of total health? Does this person understand the rest of the body? What is their evidence? Can they share the evidence for this not being good for your diabetes, or cardiovascular disease, thyroid disease, your autoimmune condition, your neurological condition? Do they understand the breadth of research that promotes overall health?" In the case of cutting out oil, for example, the target audience might be someone experiencing issues with cardiovascular health. If that's not something you're struggling with, is it the best choice for you?

"Somebody who is ethical and really understands the nuance of health will never tell you that they are going to cure you," Dahlia explained. "I never tell my patients I'm going to cure them or they are going to get better on this program. I say, 'It might work for you, it might not. I'm happy to join you on this journey and we can tweak it as we need to tweak it for you. And it might not be the thing for you at the end of the day. Because that is how our health works.'"

Back in college, I was unaware of the ways that my desire for a cure clouded my ability to think critically about the sources of my information. I decided to avoid oil for a little while and see what happened, like a cleanse. It was easy enough. I started cooking my vegetables in just a little bit of water. For dinner, I would cut up a zucchini or red cabbage, put the pieces in a pan, and let them simmer until they were mush. Salt, though against 30BaD rules, became my best friend; the food needed some sort of flavor. My dinners were no longer filling or tasty, but the sense of power I felt making a decision that might heal me made up for it.

* * *

If Durianrider's content stoked the fears I had around food, Freelee served as an example of what I thought I most wanted. When I think back to Freelee's videos now, I remember the era where a voice with a synthetic echo chanted "Raw (raw raw raw) Fit (fit fit fit) Bitch (bitch bitch bitch)," while an electronic beat pulsed in the background. My screen would turn the pale yellow of banana skin. "30 Bananas a Day, the high-carb raw vegan lifestyle" flashed by before a picture of Freelee appeared on screen. She wore a black sports bra with yellow trim and "30 Bananas a Day" emblazoned across her chest, black gloves, a black baseball cap, and low-rise leggings that featured bananas flanking her hip bones. Her stomach was flat and contoured with the suggestion of a six-pack, and she looked at the camera with a knowing grin. "Freelee TV: The Raw Fit Bitch" appeared beside her before the screen shifted just once more to her slogan: GO FRUIT YOURSELF!

This wasn't how she started out on YouTube. Her first videos, the ones I pored over while seeking a solution for my symptoms, have no flashy introduction or good lighting or really anything polished about them. Sometimes the camera isn't even focused properly on a subject. In one of her first, she says hello to the camera before panning to an array of fruit organized on a rug made of natural fibers. There are pink dragonfruit ("just sweet enough"), pineapple ("check out the beautiful color on that, I think I'm in love"), bananas ("I'm in love with bananas as well, but who isn't, hey?"), and a collection of green mangoes, red bell peppers, and zucchini to make a mango salad. She takes the viewer outside, where she's housesitting, to see the backyard. The camera shakes with the movement of her walking, and then the screen is saturated with green leaves. "This is sweet leaf and this is how easy it is to pick, harvest," she says, and she gently pinches her fingers around a single stalk, collecting all the leaves in a neat bundle as she slides her hand down. The video offers a kind of closeness; it's just her and the camera. Her voice, as a few commenters note below the video, almost sounds shy. Back in my loneliest moments, the setup of the camera made it feel as if she were my friend. I could escape from my apartment and be whisked away to a different house, to a different life. I could imagine myself as someone who might eat a pile of tropical fruit for breakfast, find greens from a nearby tree, and feel at peace. If I were more like Freelee, I might love my body.

On a granular level, a video like the one I've described, "How much fruit I eat in a day on Go Fruit Yourself," doesn't seem negative. It's simply one person telling a camera about her particular eating habits and using language like "beautiful" to describe fruit piled up on a jute rug. In some ways, it's a delightful use of the internet; Freelee's video offered me connection to someone literally halfway around the world, who ate in a way I hadn't heard of before following her. Her video felt—and still feels—like a friend inviting you into their house to see their fridge or pantry, a form of intimacy we're rarely granted in real life. What we eat can be so personal, revealing not only preferences, but also class, culture, access to food sources, dietary restrictions, and the influences of greater structures like religious or ethical beliefs that might guide our choices. Disclosing eating habits to other people—through a pantry tour, sharing a meal, or online—can be a form of vulnerability or an invitation to connect. That suddenly I was able to access that kind of closeness via the internet seemed revelatory.

I wasn't the only one who found daily vlogs of food intake alluring. "What I eat in a day" videos, as they've come to be called, originated in the early 2010s. Christine (Davidsson) Sandal, in her thesis, "You are what you eat online," cites a video, "What I Eat in a Day on 80/10/10," published on January 7, 2010, by a thin, blond woman with the username rawsynergytv as one of the first, whereas an article on *Refinery29* credits both Freelee The Banana Girl and FullyRaw Kristina (another prominent raw fruit eater) as creating some of the first in 2011 and 2012. In the years since, the genre has exploded in popularity and expanded from YouTube alone to variations on TikTok and Instagram. Everyone from vegans to carnivores to nutritionists on social media has pulled together curated footage of the food they ate in a day, but the genre was originally heavily saturated with vegan—particularly high-carb, low-fat, raw vegan—creators sharing how exactly they attained over 2,000 calories on mainly fruit.

Part of this was practical, just a modern-day variation of a sample menu in a diet book. If you told someone to "just eat fruit," you'd probably get questions like: How much? Only fruit? Are there recipes you follow or do you literally just pick up an apple? In Essie Honiball's memoir, for example, she answers questions posed to her from 1958 to 1973, including, "Do you mix fruit?" "How often do you eat?" "How and where do I eat my fruit meals?" "How much do I eat every day?" And, the age-old question that every vegan probably tires of, "Where do I get my protein?" Because she didn't have YouTube or Instagram to disseminate information to hundreds or thousands of people at once,

Essie took to the page. She went as far as to list out specifically what she ate on days one through three after completing a fast (yes to fresh fruit, no to any beverage but water with a "dash of lemon") and emphasized that people should eat exclusively one type of fruit for around a week (she chooses grapes all week long, as an example). Arnold Ehret, the one who claimed that fasting and fruit healed him of Bright's disease, in his 1924 book *Professor Arnold Ehret's Mucusless Diet Healing System*, reminded readers that "the ideal and most natural method of eating is the mono-diet. One kind of fresh fruit, when in season, should constitute a meal." If that wasn't available, he suggested what a day of eating might look like:

> Baked Apple with Honey.
> Elimination Salad.
> Baked Artichoke.
> Zweibach

(The "Elimination Salad" has more appetizing ingredients than its name might suggest: spinach, coleslaw, green peas, celery, lemon juice, and oil.) To look at sample menus through rose-colored glasses might mean saying that these types of diet books—and subsequently "What I eat in a day" videos—offer people an option beyond their own current reality and an invitation to try new foods, different recipes, or simply become aware of eating habits outside of their own. However, like anything, there is a dark side.

Take the books, for example. Arnold Ehret intentionally adds "Professor" to the title of his, making himself seem more credible (he was an art professor, not a trained nutritionist). For some people, he is regarded as a visionary, the "original father of naturopathy"—curiously enough, his book is what drew Steve Jobs to fruitarianism—but he also spouted some wild, unverified claims. He was deeply obsessed with constipation and, like Cornelius, with the idea that if you ate incorrectly and got ill, it was your fault that you had turned yourself into a "living cesspool." In his book, he writes about autopsy experts who told him about "worms and decades-old feces-stones" and notes that he has had patients eliminate "as much as 50 to 60 pounds waste, and 10 to 15 pounds alone from the colon, mainly consisting of foreign matters." (Is this sounding like a late-night infomercial yet?) Like any good grifter, he came up with a solution to relieve people of the "unknown, decayed and fermented mass of matter in the human body, decades old—especially in the intestines and colon." He started selling a laxative called INNER-CLEAN that he advertised would "scour the Intestines as Effectively as a Brush." Scour it did. After one woman consulted her physician relative to ask if there were particles of glass in the product, the Chemical Laboratory of the American Medical Association (AMA) discovered the laxatives were just a mix of "chopped-up herbs, mainly senna" and some sand. In 1926, *The Journal of the AMA* published a scathing review that the laxative was so harmful "even intelligent laymen" would notice. Did this stop Arnold Ehret? Definitely not. Brazen enough to send along a pamphlet for his *Mucusless-Diet Healing System* book as an ad with the laxatives, he continued gaining followers. Even as of 2020, there is a Facebook group dedicated to his methodologies, with someone commenting, "How can I get the innerclean that Professor Arnold Ehret recommends?"

Historically, as Christine Sandal notes in her thesis, advice dispensed from experts (or at least people in positions of authority) was taken more seriously than that of a peer. Technology hasn't changed many of the core tenets of the ideas distributed to the public—fatphobia, racism, ableism, and unverified health claims still run rampant, as does productive dialogue about food shared cross-culturally or intergenerationally—but it has changed the nature of the way this information is shared. When Arnold Ehret, Essie Honiball, and others were sharing their ideas via books, communication with practitioners was slower. It involved letters sent via mail, sometimes internationally. It meant traveling to attend a talk, which sometimes because of cost and distance simply wasn't feasible. With a vlog, that distance is erased, at least in some ways. Followers can comment on a YouTube video, ask questions via Instagram, send an email in just a few minutes. As Sandal notes, vlogging daily eats is a mashup of the "unscripted" nature of reality TV, a cooking show, and cookbooks, as the person in front of the camera usually delivers information about food or recipes while "seemingly giv[ing] access to the backstage of who someone 'really' is." Unlike in the past, when figures in authority would dole out information from a place of knowing more than others, vlogging allows for the illusion of peer-to-peer contact, meaning that parasocial relationships and platform are imperative. If a person wants to influence, Sandal notes, they must create "an active public persona" and "stress their distinctiveness, while simultaneously insinuating that there's no distinction . . . giving the illusion of individual choice." In Freelee's case, this meant selling the idea that she was different from other fitness gurus who might tell you to starve yourself, take pills, fast, or exercise to the point of exhaustion to lose weight. She was giving you the most natural diet available, free from toxins, additives, fat, and everything else that might hold you back from being your most energized, beautiful self. The loophole that set her eating plan apart from other diets was that you could—and should—be eating as much as you want, absolutely smashing in the fruit, so long as it was pure.

*   *   *

Freelee's emphasis on clean eating was what first drew former follower Lauren Coleman to the lifestyle. Coleman grew up surrounded by her mom's collection of diet books and trashy magazines replete with diet plans; she read them all. One book in particular, *Skinny Bitch*, seemed on the surface like it would be a helpful weight loss guide, but it turned out to make quite an ethical case for veganism. Coleman was intrigued by claims that eating a vegan diet would naturally be higher in fiber, lower in fat, and therefore more nutritional, but the book left her with no real idea of how to start. She purchased a stack of vegan cookbooks that led to her eating dishes heavy on soaked, blended cashews, and she found that she spent all her time preparing meals but was still hungry afterward. It was then that she found Freelee, whose content resonated with her because she urged followers not to fear carbs, to eat 2,000 to even 3,000 calories a day, and to keep fat intake super low.

"I was an impressionable twenty-year-old who was obsessed with health. I wanted the perfect body as well. The fact that Freelee was always walking around in a crop top and booty shorts, she looked amazing," Coleman reflected in a 2021 interview over Zoom. "I wanted to be like her." Unlike the vagueness Coleman found in the pages of other diet books, Freelee showed her through "What I eat in a day" videos exactly how and what to eat, and explained why certain foods, like oil, were completely off-limits. "It just seemed to make sense," Coleman expressed. "Why would you not eat food that's full of life, that's so fresh? You believed that there was something about eating this much fruit that was going to invigorate your cells and be almost as close to a spiritual awakening as possible, through a diet."

While the diet sounded romantic, the reality for Coleman was not. At the time she started eating a high-carb, low-fat, raw vegan diet, she was working twelve to fourteen hours a day at a pizza restaurant. On good days, she would blend up bananas at home and bring her smoothie to work in a giant bottle, sipping from it all day. On days she didn't have time to make a smoothie, she would go to a local fruit and veggie store nearby (she was cautious about shopping at the larger supermarket in the area because Freelee had warned followers about eating unripe bananas, which is what they tended to carry) and try to find the spottiest bananas. If those were unavailable, she would return to the pizza shop carrying a box of Medjool dates or grapes. Some days, she would stuff her backpack full of bananas and eat them the entire day. Even though sometimes it felt impractical, she stuck with it. She believed she was doing something good for herself. "I had a feeling of superiority," Coleman said. "My body was so clean."

Coleman's emphasis on purity soon extended from Freelee's teachings to other beliefs about food. She was skeptical of canned food because she had heard from other sources that they had too much BPA, which would negatively impact her endocrine system. She was scared of eating vegan protein like tofu. She refused to add peanut butter or chopped up nuts to her oatmeal, as she considered them to be too fatty. Even when her teeth began to hurt on the fruit diet, even when she began to experience energy crashes that left her wanting to stay in bed all day, even when she grew tired of stuffing the calories in for an hour or so each meal, she kept trying to follow Freelee's teachings. Coleman began to feel trapped—her food could never be pure enough, and even if she did eat the cleanest diet she could, she was left feeling bloated, tired, and unsatisfied, not to mention she was shelling out more money than she might have liked for the most organic, ripest sources of fruit. When she finally reached her tipping point, she fell into a cycle of eating "clean" and then bingeing on pizza and chocolate other days. Still chasing the elusive idea of the perfect diet, she did not immediately find balance.

What Coleman and others experienced while pursuing a high-carb, raw vegan diet aligns with the very premise of naturopathy, which emphasizes that an individual's system is capable of ridding itself of toxins if it is not overwhelmed by too much food or the wrong kinds of food, as long as a person is given small doses of sunlight, a place to bathe, and regular exercise. Naturopathy emphasizes individualism and self-reliance; your body can heal itself, so long as you treat it the right way. There's nothing inherently wrong with naturopathy itself, or the idea of alternative cures, but believing that methods like fasting, procuring doses of sunlight, or eating monomeals of a certain fruit will heal you from all ills (everything from gout to demons to toxins to cancer) can be dangerous. Without any credible nutritional study attached, these rules make it so practitioners carry the burden of ensuring they remain "pure" enough for the diet to work. If a diet based on naturopathic ideas fails, it can easily be blamed on the individual (e.g., "You have acne because you combined mangoes and bananas") rather than the system itself.

This is a tale as old as time—or at least as old as Essie and Cornelius, Arnold Ehret, Johanna Brandt, and all the practitioners of purity who came before. Brandt claimed that grapes could free "the blood from gouty and rheumatic poisons," dissolve and expel "inorganic deposits that have settled between the joints" through "diarrhea or an unpleasant oily sweat," and cause appendicitis to "lose its terrors." She viewed grapes as something of an almighty cleanse, one that could cure a person instantly.

Ehret, in his *Mucusless Diet Healing System*, insists that fruit and greens are the only "right" food, which he knows not through scientific testing, but because God declared it so in Genesis 1:29. Ehret thought that doctors intentionally told their patients to eat "destructive foods" so that they would stay in business, said that people all had the power to be disease-free if only they followed his dietary suggestions. He believed that if a child was born ill, it was because of the combination of a "filthy, mostly constipated colon and an unclean bladder of a civilized mother." Women, he believed, should aspire to "Madonna-like, holy purity" by getting rid of the "monthly flow of impure blood and other waste." Most alarmingly, though we would label this as amenorrhea now and consider it cause for a nutritional and/or mental health intervention of some sort, Ehret bragged that "every one of my female patients reported their menses as becoming less and less, then a two, three and four months' intermission, and finally entirely disappearing."

As for Essie, she says that Cornelius and those who came before him referred to any food that wasn't fruit as "poisons," "impurities," "mucus," "incorrect eating," "pollution," and "contamination." Eating the "wrong" foods, according to Cornelius and Essie, would cause disease, degeneration, ugliness, decay, and death.

But even eating the "right" foods didn't bring people immediate relief. Instead, Essie writes in her memoir that when she first started the fruit diet, she remembers fainting two or three times on her way from the bathroom to the bedroom because she was so weak from hunger. She only continued because the weakness was a sign she was "purging" herself of "harmful substances." The thin line between health and death that exists when people are urged into disordered eating—or take up fasting—is alarming, particularly when symptoms like weakness, fainting, sweating, etc. are labeled as proof that the cure is working, rather than as a body's cry for help. Even at Essie's happiest, when she was visiting different fruit orchards in the VW van, she was tested by hunger and by cravings for the foods of her past. With Cornelius by her side, she was strong enough to overcome the challenges brought on by the diet, but not long after the pair returned to civilization, Cornelius took a fall and experienced hemorrhaging in his brain. Before he passed, he told Essie to stay true to fruit. His last words to her: "See how far you can go and how high you can aim."

Essie tried her best to stay on the right path while remaining part of society, but she no longer had Cornelius's "honesty, courage, determination, serenity and mental clarity" to guide her. She attended dinner parties with old friends and new colleagues but refused every dish and drink that the host might offer. As Anoeschka von Meck, Essie's South African biographer, explained to me in an interview, Essie's reluctance to partake in refreshments at parties would not have been seen as her being just impolite. Instead, in South Africa during that time period, especially in the rural towns where Essie lived, hospitality was a form of love and care, a way of forging and maintaining relationships with other people. For Essie to deny not only refreshments like tea, coffee, or biscuits, but also more significant items like meat, would have been a rejection of her community's values, their culture, and most of all, their friendship. They stopped inviting her to gatherings and parties. Friends, scientists, and doctors alike all told Essie that her new way of eating was "evil." They warned her that her bones would decalcify. They told her she would be deficient in nutrients. They told her to abandon her "crazy diet" before it was too late.

It wasn't long before Essie's daily life was characterized by isolation. And in her loneliness, she became extremely anxious. Cornelius was a great love of her life, someone who had saved her from the most dire of circumstances. How could she stay true to what he wanted for her when it led to so much additional pain? Without him, she had no one to buffer the waves of rejection she felt in so many social encounters, no one to remind her why eating fruit was the only way she could heal herself from the ills of the world. Her cravings for comfort became so strong that she began slipping. She remembers eating potatoes. In her memoir she writes, "My willpower had disappeared like mist before the sun and I sat eating potatoes like an alcoholic enslaved by drink. After two days of eating potatoes, my tongue turned bright blue and stung so much that I could eat nothing, not even potatoes." To quell her cravings, she went alone to the top of a mountain with a basket of fruit and stayed there for a few days. There, removed from society and from temptation, she was "once again ready to continue [her] pilgrimage" as a fruit-eater and purify her body once more.

* * *

Early in her fruit journey, Freelee was scared enough of the toxic metals in blenders that she smashed fruit by hand to make smoothies. When Douglas Graham brought tahini to one of his seminars, Freelee and Durianrider were taken aback. *Is it pure?* they wondered. *Is it certifiably raw?* I listened to Freelee and Durianrider preach about the importance of a particular kind of health in their YouTube videos and read enough of the online 30BaD forum that their emphasis on purity seeped into my life in a way that seemed innocent at first. On my weekly trip to the grocery store with roommates, I picked up oatmeal for breakfast and added extra fruits and veggies to my cart. I decided I would get rid of "bad" food: olive oil, peanut butter, Earth Balance, pasta, baked goods, and meat. I figured, if anything, that eating a diet higher in carbs and lower in fat might show me proof that the method worked. If it did, then maybe I'd be convinced to try an even cleaner diet of fruit and only fruit.

When I prepared my oatmeal in the microwave each morning, I told myself that I didn't need to add almond milk; water was good enough, more hydrating. As much as I wanted a dollop of nut butter on top or a drizzle of honey to sweeten things up, I reminded myself that fat would harm me. I tried to keep the food as plain as possible for easy digestion. For lunch, I usually ate a big salad—spinach, chopped cucumbers, cherry tomatoes, bell peppers, and sometimes a handful of garbanzo beans. I'd either eat the salad raw or pour just a touch of balsamic vinegar on top. Dinner was the most difficult meal, only because I couldn't be alone to eat whatever low-fat, low-calorie, plant-based creation I had devised to suit my ever-increasing list of fear foods. Like Lauren Coleman, I had started to believe that fat was poison. Sometimes, I would team up with Andrea to make spaghetti squash in the oven, convincing her that we could use a splash of water on both halves rather than the olive oil we typically drizzled on it.

It helped that Andrea was vegan to begin with, so she never questioned my desire to abstain from certain foods, but my immersion into 30BaD also came at a time when, culturally, there were more examples of the 30BaD-type lifestyle, even if it wasn't explicitly labeled as such. Rip Esselstyn, a blue-eyed firefighter from Austin, Texas, had recently come out with a book called *The Engine 2 Diet* in which he stressed the importance of eating a plant-based, oil-free diet. He was commercially successful enough to quit his firefighting job and partner with Whole Foods, where he sold a line of Engine 2 Plant-Strong foods like broths, granola, frozen meals, and cereal that didn't include the "off-limits" ingredients outlined in his book. His feature on *Forks Over Knives* and easy-to-access online recipes meant that when I made his oil-free plant-based lasagna for my roommates one night, it afforded us all a chance to share a meal.

If I ever fell prey to a bite of chocolate chip cookie dough when my roommates made it, I'd chew for just a few moments, torn between pleasure and guilt all the while, before secretly spitting the half-masticated ball into a sink. Instead of joining in our apartment dinners with the full vigor and closeness I had in the past, I often sat on the sidelines eating the rubbery no-carb noodles that come in a plastic bag. I was perpetually in a state of anxiety about how I would participate in group events while not saying out loud what I had begun to believe. My fears around food began to intersect with the terror I experienced living in my own uncontrollable body. Though the quantity of my episodes had diminished greatly in the weeks since my mom had left campus, if I became episodic, I blamed some facet of my nutrition first.

During those weeks, I summited a lonely mountain of my own. Despite the discomfort I felt—the hunger, the cravings, the distance from my friends—I now understand why Essie and others didn't leave the fruit lifestyle behind, and why I had a hard time reaching for real healing. When you're in that state of mind, fear is a primary motivator. Afraid enough of returning to the darkest place you've ever been, where your body is almost unknowable to you, moralizing food gives you the illusion of safety. A guide or a guru whispering about evil versus good seems less ludicrous and more like a secret that only you are lucky enough to hear. As I waited for a bed in the epilepsy unit to open, I felt power over how much I ate and what I abstained from, and the willpower it took me to do so.

CHAPTER 17

Salvation, Starvation

THE WAY I WITHHELD FOOD FROM MYSELF DURING JUNIOR
year of college was not my first dalliance with disordered eating. My
family moved around quite a bit when I was a child, usually every
two years. Despite a propensity toward introversion (you were likely
to find me sitting in the neighborhood library reading *The Hardy Boys*
for hours alone while my brother took off on his scooter and climbed
trees with other kids outside), I had always managed to make friends.
It all seemed to change at my international school in Indonesia, when
I skipped fifth grade and moved up to sixth. On back-to-school night,
I remember walking into my new classroom. The teacher asked me for
my name. My throat constricted. I could not speak. My mom gently
prodded me in the back to make sure I had heard. "Jacqueline," I
whispered. My mom repeated my name and then gave me a glance as
if to say, *What is going on?*

The acute shyness I felt that night faded away, but I still felt like I
was out of place in my new grade. The language my peers spoke was full
of nuance. Unlike in elementary school, where I had asked boys I liked
to dance or invited a lonely girl from my class to come slide with me

and my group of friends, I could not keep up with the furtive glances, the way casual hangouts after school determined the social order within, and the comfort others seemed to have in their bodies. It only got worse in seventh grade, when we moved again, this time to Jakarta, and I showed up to my bus stop for the first day. I took care picking out my outfit: new white sneakers and a pair of overalls. When I stepped up to board the bus, a girl with blond curly hair sneered, "The elementary bus comes later," and I found myself stammering that I, in fact, was her new classmate. It was only then that I saw myself as she must have: I had a pink Igloo cooler lunchbox strapped across my shoulder, a euphonium behind me that I had rigged to a metal suitcase roller with some bungee cords, blue wire-frame glasses, and braces on my teeth. Things didn't improve much as middle school went on. I remember taking a drama class and being assigned to perform a two-person improv skit where each of us was supposed to introduce a line of dialogue and rachet up from there. Getting up in front of my classmates was always my worst nightmare, but that day, they laughed. Maybe my jokes about ants were funny? I continued with my observations of imaginary insects on a picnic blanket, and my peers kept laughing. It was only later that someone told me everyone had seen the sheen of my leg hair luminescent under the stage lights and were giggling because I hadn't yet started shaving like everyone else.

During those years, as is the case for many preteens, my body was my worst enemy. It felt impossible to wrangle. My hair curled in the equatorial humidity, I started my period, and my only interaction with boys was in my notebook, where I made comparison charts between two crushes who I don't think knew my name. I wanted to be desired—to be desirable—and I soon began to view thinness as a means to achieve that. I remember dancing in my room alone after reading in *Seventeen* that thirty minutes of dancing would burn off a burger, even though I hadn't eaten a burger for months. In the cafeteria, I would order a chicken bowl, pick off the chicken, and eat a small portion of the white, plain rice that remained. At dinners, claiming I didn't like meat very much, I would eat mango or whatever fruit we had around. Between swimming competitively during that time and going through frequent growth spurts, I soon could see my hip bones. When a mom at a swim meet told me I looked "svelte" in my suit, I beamed. In PE while changing one day, a popular girl came up to me while I had my shirt off and said, "You could be a back model." Imposing my own insecurities on her comment, I took what she said to mean I had an ugly face but that the boniness of my body redeemed me somehow.

Something about moving again—this time at the beginning of high school, to Texas—broke the rituals I had created around food. Returning to the United States after six years away meant I was dazzled by the array of chip options gleaming in gas stations, Papa John's pizza with garlic dipping sauce, and gelato I loved so much that I asked for a party tray as a reward if I did well in a regional race. By the time I got to college, I ate more than almost anyone on the team. I ate cereal before practice, deli sandwiches for lunch, and healthy servings of dinner. With a rigorous routine of running, weightlifting, and class, I was always ravenous. Plus, something about being so close to other people experiencing disordered eating—someone who just ate iceberg lettuce with a teaspoon of mustard on top, someone else who would measure out portions and do extra ab exercises on the concrete outside our dorm before allowing herself to eat—served as a reminder of the way I had punished my own body in the past. I didn't want to do that again. But when I found myself stuck in my apartment room just a couple years later, my fears surrounding food and weight gain reemerged. I don't know if it was that I was more sedentary than I had been in the past (and therefore, in some warped part of my mind, less deserving of food), or if it was the memory of an obsessive teammate asking me, "Are you going to eat that *whole* bagel?" during my first year of college, or if it was hearing my vegan roommates talking with such sureness about meat causing cancer and other health problems, but I started to wonder if somehow my intake of food had made me sick. This fear of food—whether or not I was eating the "right" thing—intersected in a dangerous way with my own perception of desirability, or lack thereof.

*   *   *

My wheelchair, a helpful device in so many ways, made each entrance feel like the one I'd made with the lunchbox and euphonium. On my own, I did not make the associations between these objects and shame, but the way that other people in the world interacted with them—and subsequently me—made me feel as though I were an outsider in spaces where I thought I wanted to belong. To get to school in those weeks, Andrea would push me across the parking lot of our apartment complex and along the red-bricked paths of campus. After being inside for so many hours alone, getting outside felt like relief. There was a sky, big and blue above me. A breeze that teased at my hair. Trees and squirrels and the marginalia of conversations as people passed us by. Movement forward. The embarrassment came when we got inside. Andrea would bring me into an elevator and we would disembark at the top floor. My cheeks grew heated whenever we rolled into class. I had no boot on my foot or wrap around my knee or any other physical marker as a reason to use a wheelchair. Andrea would pull a desk out of the way, push me to the empty spot she had made in the front row, and then leave me so she could attend her own class.

Those minutes, while everyone trickled in, were the most painful. I would reach slowly into my backpack and take as long as I could to retrieve the one notebook I carried with me. I studied the back cover of the anthology we read from as if it were an indecipherable map and counted down the minutes until class began. I'd had the professor, Dr. Schwind, the year before. On the first day of the previous semester's course, she had announced to us that she wore hearing aids. If she didn't respond to the sound of our voices, it simply meant she hadn't heard us or could not see that we were speaking. She was very matter of fact in explaining her disability. I think that some part of me knew, because of this, that she might be more empathetic toward my situation than other educators I had encountered who, due to my appearance as a person with no quantifiable features of illness, were curt with me or downright dismissive when I tried discussing accommodations.

During freshman year, for example, when I told one professor that I had been released from the ER with neurological issues the night before, she responded that if I was capable of walking, I should be in class. At that point, believing I should—and could—overcome any physical discomfort, I left thirty minutes early to traverse a quarter of a mile. In class, my head rocked and my vision blurred to the point that I couldn't see the board or the pages in front of me. My notes from that day read, in part: "I mean both I mean very very smart Romans no knows about Romans . . . well um um this lady um oh writer yeah she was um um the well first yeah lady writer early travel writer yeah what?" Other professors commented that I should speak up more in class, and I did not yet have the language to explain that my silence wasn't borne out of a lack of interest, but a fear of becoming episodic mid-sentence.

In Dr. Schwind's class, all my peers were kind enough—no one ever made a rude remark or asked me any uncomfortable questions— but seeing them in such close proximity reminded me I was missing out. Addressing one another, they lobbed questions about upcoming tests, rehashed parties, and invited each other to intramural teams. Aside from chiming into class discussions on occasion, I didn't really talk to anyone, as I was terrified that my words would melt into something incoherent. And what did I have to offer even if I could speak? A botched study-abroad trip, hours spent alone in my room browsing through obscure corners of the internet, my name on a waiting list for the epilepsy unit. In those moments, I felt so disconnected from the life of a college student, it was as if I were wandering down the empty halls of an old home I'd once lived in. The space echoed with reminders of who I might have been had I not collapsed that first time on a track. I might have been a little more confident, made friends outside my apartment, gone to a party, or driven down the farmland roads just for fun, with my windows down and the radio all the way up. I might have trusted that many people were inherently good rather than assessing them for potential risk. Riddled still with the unresolved memory of my teammate pressing me down to my mattress and taunted still by the echoes of *freak* and *whale*, I shied away from contact with anyone new, especially men.

But there was one guy in class, I'll call him Ben, who was mild-mannered and quiet compared to his group of friends. Because of the travel chair, I stuck out into the front aisle of the classroom and no one occupied the seats next to me. Each day, Ben would nod hello, carefully maneuver past my backpack, and then take up a seat just a couple back from me. When he raised his hand to speak in class, which was rare, his words carried the hint of a stutter. I liked this about him. My cheeks grew warm when he would slide past me at the end of class, always with such attention to the contours of my frame, and I found myself trying to suppress feelings of giddiness that rose within me whenever he was around. I wasn't allowed to have a crush, I told myself. At that point, I had convinced myself of my own undesirability. Not even *I* liked my body, so why would anyone else? I had seen what men did to me when I was incoherent; I wouldn't risk that again. But one day, when everyone had left the classroom and I was stuck waiting for Andrea, Ben asked me if I'd like him to push me somewhere. I could tell, from his stammer and the blush in his cheeks, that it had taken him courage to ask. I could tell, from the way he stood with his hands gently curled, that he would have pushed me anywhere, with no threat of malice. I was so ashamed of myself at that moment, so infuriated that I couldn't have the chance to know him in a body that felt more like mine, that I quickly said no. Then, as he walked away, I felt the sudden urge to cry.

*   *   *

When Andrea dropped me back at the apartment that day, I had a few hours to while away before everyone returned home. My phone was mostly a reminder of my parents calling to see how I was (I often lied and responded that I was doing fine) or to ask me if I had heard from Duke about my upcoming stay, which I hadn't. As much as I could, I avoided thinking about the hospital. I was at odds with the idea of a diagnosis. Part of me thought I might feel relief if given a name for what I had experienced, that I might finally feel like what I had gone through had been real. But the other part of me feared what a diagnosis would really mean. Whenever I had brought up the word "epilepsy" in the past, people had reacted with a kind of fearful, faraway look that indicated their discomfort, as well as mine. Would it be something I would have to disclose to others? To future employers? Would I have to be medicated? What might it look like to have a relationship? Would I have to live in that bleary, foggy place that the anti-seizure medication had taken me to forever? There was also the chance that, in the hospital, there would be no diagnosis, no answers. I didn't even know how to reckon with that kind of uncertainty or think about the ways that a diagnosis *(or lack of one) might impact my perception of self. I didn't turn to any of my usual coping mechanisms—running far or talking to Eliza—to process the upcoming hospital stay and the ways that I felt stymied by my health. Instead, I chose to numb myself by turning to the place that had begun to bring me comfort: Freelee's YouTube channel.

At the time I was watching, in 2012, Freelee's header was a bright yellow, featuring text that read "Freelee TV: The Raw Fit Bitch." I remember watching the videos for the monotony; I could lose myself in the routine of Freelee eating massive quantities of fruit for breakfast, lunch, and dinner. But looking back at her channel, I realize I was also drawn in by the way her body was used as a message: Eat fruit and you can have the body of your dreams. Speckled cartoon bananas, a pair of pink undies with "30 Bananas a Day" emblazoned on the back, and "My Before & Afters" featuring mirrored images of Freelee's face populated the top of the screen. There was sex appeal laced through the front page, too: Freelee in lingerie next to "Raw Food Videos every MONDAY"; Freelee mid-strip, revealing low-cut underwear and a black bra; a video titled "Raw Food Vegan SEX" featuring a thumbnail of Durianrider biting into a banana while Freelee looks on; Freelee, clad in strappy black bikini underwear and a black bra, "Sexy dancing fruitarian girl in underwear"; Freelee wearing "Sexy Halloween Fruit Dresses" in front of her unmade bed. The titles might offer a glimpse into Freelee's and Durianrider's mindsets while building their platforms, as they have since been tamed to more accurately represent the content featured. (For example, the video "Raw Food Vegan SEX" is now labeled "Raw Food Vegan Advice" and "Sexy dancing fruitarian girl in underwear" is now "Freelee having fun.") This early glimpse at Freelee's YouTube also shows how much her body was featured in comparison to the fruit. The rhetorical message sent through these thumbnails is that a banana smoothie might not be as appetizing as the promise of a striptease.

Freelee using sex appeal to sell a diet isn't news; look at any billboard, pop-up ad, or commercial of a woman launching herself happily through the air after eating a light yogurt, and you'll see many of the same techniques used. What is interesting, though, is that while Freelee was using sexualized images of herself to promote her way of life, she was also rejecting what she termed "the system." In a video, "How to become a SLAVE to the system," Freelee sits next to her bed and what looks to be a potted peace lily. She's wearing lingerie covered by a loosely knitted mesh cover-up, and she takes on a voice that sounds like a flight attendant giving instructions. She explains "how to become a mindless drone," telling viewers sarcastically to "get a huge mortgage that will take you the next fifty years to pay off," go out with friends to a pub, "wake up with a nasty hangover and risk facing reality," before going out to a "breakfast binge-out" to eat food like "milkshakes, cheese, bacon, eggs . . . the best mind-numbing foods" that she says will totally wreck your adrenals. What Freelee does, in this video and others, is set up a false equivalency between fruit eating and lifestyle that extends far beyond eating habits themselves. (Choosing a diet other than exclusively fruit does not necessarily mean you'll wake up and drink a milkshake every morning, hate your job, and generally be miserable.) As Christine Sandal writes, "categories of clean and unclean are highly symbolic, as there is no universal 'truth' behind them, but they rather signify a desire to maintain order." This order not only applies to what food people put on their plates, but also extends to other areas of life, where the onus is placed on individuals to make decisions that give them "good health, a good body shape, and a happy life."

While I'd like to say I was able to see through the ways Freelee moralized food and lifestyle decisions at the time I was first watching her videos, I can't. So much of the rhetoric she used to describe "good" decisions versus "bad" ones correlated with my own internal dialogue at the time. I was bad because I couldn't run, bad because I wasn't sick enough to have a diagnosis but also bad because I was symptomatic enough to be in a wheelchair, bad because I couldn't will my body into submission the way that I thought I should be able to. Winnowing my body into something smaller seemed to be the only way for me to express, at least outwardly, some measure of control over my form, so I kept listening to Freelee. In her videos, often while wearing a cropped green "Go Fruit Yourself" T-shirt and low-rise, hip-hugging leggings, she ranted about how messed up our society was for preaching calorie restriction; she wanted people to enjoy an abundance of fruit. She talked about how far she could ride on her bike, how much endurance and energy stemmed from her diet. She told me about how I could heal myself by heading to a mono-fruit island.

Taking up a totally fruit-based diet would mean giving up the indulgences I had allowed myself, like carrots dipped into salsa, popcorn made in the microwave with no oil, or squash covered in low-fat marinara sauce. I figured I owed it to myself to try. I pitched it to Andrea as an experiment of sorts, and we got so into it that she donned a pair of oversized reading glasses, pulled out a large Five Star notebook, and pretended to be my psychiatrist for the day. (Whether or not she was actually worried for my mental health at that point is something I haven't asked her, but I can imagine that she might have been.) I began the day with a mono-meal of bananas and ate just a couple; I didn't know how my body would react to too much fruit and figured, based on the recent paltry portions I had been serving myself, that it would keep me full until lunch. At midday, I ate a handful of grapes, and by mid-afternoon I remember curling into our armchair and whining to Andrea about how hungry I was. She pushed her glasses down her nose and, in her best therapist voice, said, "Tell me more about that." By night, it was as much a feeling of wanting to rebel against a set of rules I hadn't created as it was hunger that led me to cut a cucumber and sprinkle it with so much salt that I declared I was eating an ocean. After that came sweet potatoes sliced up and baked on a cookie sheet. I had broken down after not even a full day of fruitarianism, which maybe was as much psychological as physical. If I adopted a wholly fruitarian diet and it *still* didn't work, then what would that say about my body? I might feel even more defective.

* * *

In addition to sex appeal, Freelee put thinness at the forefront of her messaging. In her e-book *Go Fruit Yourself,* Freelee emphasizes her own weight loss while talking about how eating a high-carb, raw vegan diet helped her heal from a history of disordered eating. "Anorexia is brought about by poor nutrition, a lack of education and an abundance of negative conditioning via mainstream media and other avenues," Freelee writes. Even in the early days of trying to heal herself from her eating disorder, Freelee struggled to know how much food was enough. Where was the line between fueling herself and bingeing? An example of this, she writes, is that in 2006, on an unnamed raw food forum, Freelee posted (under the username FREELEERAW) that she "had a little bit of an over-eating session." She had consumed three bananas in one sitting, which alarmed her. Years later, during the writing of her e-book, she reflects, "Did I overeat? Of course not. What a nut job! With all the training I was doing I was obviously not overeating. I NEEDED the fuel . . . This uneducated thought process can turn us into paranoid crazies, and I'm SO glad I have now nipped it in the butt [sic]. These days my goal is to eat as MUCH sweet fruit as I can, no more anorexic mentality. This lifestyle is all about abundance and if we are to succeed on it we must embrace this way of thinking."

While Freelee's message on the surface might seem positive (heal your-self from disordered eating and enjoy food in abundance!), it came with a stipulation: Freelee also preached an anti-fat message of attaining—and maintaining—the "perfect" physique, which, to her, apparently exclu-sively meant being slim. Rather than rejecting what was sold to her by "negative conditioning via mainstream media," the titles of Freelee's early videos (and beyond) read like the cover of a tabloid in a grocery store:

Biggest FAT LOSS fitness Secret! No gimmicks . . .
How To Get A Flat Stomach! [1 YEAR LATER UPDATE]
Raw food vegan weight loss secrets #1—The scales
Vegan for 6 years & 40 lbs. lighter!
The BEST fat-burner food is BANANAS!
5 Reasons You Are Still Fat and a semi-rant!

By Freelee's fifth video posted to YouTube, the content shifts from montages of fruit and plants to something different. In this one, in a foreboding sign of power dynamics to come, she's no longer holding the camera. Instead, she's standing in front of what looks to be a large floor-to-ceiling window in a house, one completely blackened by night. She's wearing low-rise jeans and a purple crop top that shows off her cleavage. She smiles for the camera.

"Okay, Freelee, so tell us a bit about what you ate today," Durianrider says from behind the lens.

"What did I eat today—" Freelee muses.

"Everything you ate," Durianrider interjects. "And don't leave anything out."

Freelee lists two liters of orange juice (followed by a "Yep" from Durianrider), fifteen bananas ("Yep"), another fifteen bananas for dinner, and three liters of water. The interaction begins to feel a bit like the investigation of a crime, as Durianrider badgers her with questions: "When did you drink the water?" "Why is that? Why is that?" "So you drank a liter of water before you had your orange juice?" "Are you an athlete?" "Does water help your digestion?"

Then he asks, "Can you just turn to the side for a minute, so we can see your stomach?" Freelee smiles. She turns to the side, visibly flexing her core. With her fingers hooked through her jeans, she sticks her bum out a bit and turns to look at Durianrider. "Don't suck in too much," he responds. She relaxes her posture and smiles. "That's it, just relax it." She turns for the camera like a model, posing so we can see her abs and then twirling so we get a glimpse of her whole body, as if to say, no gimmicks here, this is the real deal.

"Fruit makes you fat," she says cheekily, and Durianrider tilts the camera down so we can see her legs, and then pans back up, as if to check her out.

* * *

In many ways, I do not place personal blame on Freelee for espousing the rhetoric of "before and after" in the early days of 30BaD, or for using clickbait titles for her first YouTube videos; we are all, in different ways, still operating within the same system that led women like Lady Mary Wortley Montagu to reach for asses' milk out of desperation way before us, one that privileges thin, white bodies. Freelee, at this point in her career, probably believed that if she weaponized the allure of thinness to her advantage, she could win more people in her fight to save the animals and the planet. In many ways, it worked.

One member of 30BaD, whom I'll refer to as Jan, introduced herself on the site as a student at the University of Georgia who was interested in nutrition. Like Freelee had in her own journey, Jan also went through ups and downs with raw food. She had turned to veganism after a struggle with anorexia as a teenager, but says she wasn't "being a raw foodist in the proper way and became very sick." Her family, concerned by her decline in health, encouraged her to eat meat, dairy, and eggs again, even though Jan "had read so many books as to why these foods are unhealthy." She posted, "After about a year of gaining nearly 10 lbs and being sick with bad skin, I am ready to go back to a raw vegan lifestyle. I am in need of guidance and am in search of the best eating plan to be healthy, thin and happy!!" On October 7, 2012, Jan posted that she was starting her 30-day challenge; at 5'6", she was 128 pounds, and she wanted to lose thirteen. The questions she poses to fellow followers reveal her anxieties about her body: "Does anyone have any feedback as to how long it took for you to begin loosing [sic] weight? Did you gain any weight at first adjusting to the higher calorie intake? Do I work out before or after I've eaten? Can I eat the bananas spaced out or should I eat 10-15 in one sitting? Do HCRV [high-carb, raw vegan] people eat other fruits that aren't quite as high in carbs such as berries, apples, melon, etc.?"

She was far from the only person in her late teens to be lured in by the promise of eating abundantly while still maintaining a very thin figure. In a 2018 Reddit thread posted under r/EDAnonymous (Eating Disorders Anonymous), titled "Fuck freelee the banana girl," user crashdietdummy posted, "That woman literally started all my disordered eating and thinking. What a mess. She really had me believing that eating 3,000 calories of fruit every day would paradoxically make you both underweight and extremely healthy??? I can still hear her saying 'yoa boday runs on shoogah.'" Others related similar stories in the comments. A user named SkinnyFantasies found Freelee when they already had an eating disorder and "believed her when she said that her high calorie, high fruit/carb diet could cure my ED and at first I thought it did. I was no longer afraid of eating lots of food, but that high sugar diet gave me terrible digestion issues that have spiraled into many more health issues that I still struggle with to this day 5 years after I've stopped 'smashing in the fruit.'" And NewKid00 summed it up succinctly by reflecting, "Those were some dark days man."

By including these reflections, I am not inextricably linking disordered eating and fruitarianism or a vegan diet; for some individuals, eating a fruit-based diet brings them fulfillment and makes them feel good, and it is *very* possible to eat a well-balanced plant-based diet. However, the patterns in the questions posted to forums and even Freelee's own reckoning with quantities of food (how much fruit was enough, for example) show clearly how followers might have benefited from sessions with trained professionals, who would have scientific data to back their claims, and also be able to craft individualized nutrition plans. Additionally, the demonization of entire categories of food, like fat, begins to toe the thin line between "health" and disordered eating. In a 2018 article "Strict health-oriented eating patterns (orthorexic eating behaviours) and their connection with a vegetarian and vegan diet," authors list qualities of orthorexia as leading to "negative consequences such as malnutrition, impaired social life, deterioration of the quality of life, and well-being" because of "compulsive behaviours or mental pre-occupations with dietary choices believed to promote optimal health." The study's authors write that sometimes, "vegetarian diets may be used to legitimize food avoidance . . . and disguise restrictive eating patterns."

I am in no way saying that everyone on a fruitarian diet experiences disordered eating, but I do think it's important to consider 30BaD's audience and greater cultural context that might have impacted the way this particular diet was received by the public. Many of Freelee's followers were old enough to use the internet but too young to access resources like counseling or a dietician on their own, or perhaps didn't have the language yet to describe the pressures they were under or trauma they had experienced. Freelee's emphasis that you could overcome disordered eating *and* remain thin—a holy grail of sorts—attracted a particularly vulnerable population of people. Some of them gathered on an eating disorder forum in 2013 to talk about whether or not the diet would help them lose weight. They had usernames like skinnyunnie, skinnyminnyballet, and 79lbs. They listed their current weights and goal weights beneath each comment, sometimes crossing out the numbers on their way as a means of showing progress. They had bios like "Vegan • Ortho • High restriction • Obsessed with the '80s." A person with the username creperie commented, "There's a way to promote healthy eating, but she's doing it completely wrong . . . Apparently eating fully raw vegan will make your period stop since you won't have any toxins in your body . . . :blink: No, it's because you don't have enough nutrients to have a period lol." But someone else, a user named purgingally, lamented that she followed Freelee on "everything" and that she wished her "parents would allow me to go 100% raw. [Freelee] seems so happy thin and healthy with only fruit! THATS THE LIFE I NEED." The reality Freelee presented on the internet looked like a golden ticket to many people who were suffering in some way at home, from societal pressure to cultivate a certain figure to more specific forms of hurt.

One former follower, who wishes to remain anonymous, was looking for a way out of a difficult home life when she found Freelee in high school. "I came from a lot of family struggles," the former follower told me during a phone interview in 2020. Her turbulent home life led her to develop insomnia and a fear of sleeping, which made her less hungry than usual. It was the start of a dangerous chain of events. The insomnia, she described in an interview, "led me to weight loss, which led me to have this thing go off in my mind like, 'Wow, I can control what I look like. I can control my weight.' It led to an eating disorder." Her eating disorder was about exercising control. She described it as, "Having a sense of agency in my life. A sense of steering the ship, if only in the slightest way." She remembers waking up, skipping breakfast, running exactly ten times around the block, and then walking every aisle in the grocery store to buy ingredients that she thought were "safe" and "healthy." In the midst of her obsession with what foods were okay to eat, she found Freelee's YouTube channel.

When Freelee first flashed across her screen, this former follower wasn't fully able to trace the connections between her own struggles at home, her eating disorder, and her eventual fervor for high-carb veganism. Eventually, this former follower would collect thousands and thousands of followers of her own while preaching about the goodness of a high-carb vegan diet—through her platforms on YouTube, Instagram, and Tumblr. But at first, like me, this former follower felt like a spectator rather than a participant. Over time, Freelee's black-and-white approach to different foods lured her in more deeply. "The wholesale, extreme, 'you have to be this way, all or nothing' really adheres to the mindset of someone with disordered eating and the rules and the restrictions around it are—we enjoy that, I guess," the former follower told me over the phone in 2020. "We are looking for a way to express that discomfort in a way that can maybe seem socially acceptable and it seems like that movement almost made it okay to have rules around food. Like no oil, not because I have an eating disorder, but because I'm high-carb vegan. I think, in my experience, it delayed a lot of my full recovery from my eating disorder. I was in a state of quasi-recovery where I was still holding onto a lot of food rules that were masked by this lifestyle."

It wasn't just the food rules that appealed to this former follower or other people struggling with disordered eating, either. Part of the allure was the emphasis on Freelee's body: her flat stomach, her hip bones, her thin arms, the miracle of her forty-pound weight loss. "The way to get people in, the hook, was Freelee's body," this former follower reflected. "I think that sets up, at the start, a warped order of priorities for a lot of people who enter it, because if you're entering it for the body, you're not going to care about animals and health and helping the planet. Those things fall by the wayside. And because of that, it's not a very sustainable source of motivation." The emphasis on Freelee's body also limited diversity. This former follower reflected that the movement seemed "like a lot of white people. It didn't seem very inclusive in a sense, and it did seem like it was centered around the goal of attaining a body like Freelee. And it set up in some ways that once you did get that, your problems would be fixed and you would love yourself and feel worthy."

*   *   *

After my failed fruit day, I still kept to the other set of arbitrary rules I had created for myself—a mashup of the diet culture I had grown up with and the warnings about the dangers of fat from Freelee and Durianrider's videos. As I grew thinner and thinner, I began experiencing fewer neurological symptoms. It was exactly as Freelee and Durianrider said it would be. I started taking short walks around campus. I made my way to class alone and relished the feeling of a clear head. Like the triumphant end of a testimonial on 30BaD, I was out in the world! Moving around on my own! Meeting my roommate in the dining hall for salad! (Cue trumpets!) Though in reality I don't think that my diet had much, if anything, to do with my recovery (I think it was more a product of resting for weeks in my room and leaving the high altitude of my study abroad in Peru that did the trick), I began to equate "pure" eating with symptom-free days.

CHAPTER 13

Rebuke the Unclean Spirit

I'VE FORGOTTEN WHETHER DUKE UNIVERSITY HOSPITAL called me in North Carolina or my mom in Oklahoma to let us know that a bed would be open the next week, but I do remember receiving a large envelope in my apartment mailbox with documents relevant to my stay. Enclosed was a brochure titled something like, "How to Prepare Your Child for a Visit to the Epilepsy Center." Tacked to the front of the brochure was a Post-it Note, and on it someone had written that they knew I wasn't technically a child, but the information might come in handy. I tried making a joke to my mom over the phone about how ridiculous it was that she needed to check in with me, a twenty-year-old, to make sure I washed my hair before check-in, or the fact that I needed an "Adult Observer" to stay with me all three days, but my humor fell flat. The memory of her coaxing me to sip broth just a few months before was too fresh for us both. In a way, the brochure made real what angered me about my illness: I felt infantilized, like I wasn't capable of caring for myself or telling the doctors how I felt on my own. I was angry that I had less control than I wanted over how and when I received answers, and that I needed an "adult" to communicate information on my behalf.

In the days leading up to my mom's arrival in North Carolina, I remember walking as far as I could down the old farmland roads I had once run. The weather was slowly warming with the arrival of spring, and the trees were gaining back their green. Tied to one of the mailboxes was an *"It's a girl"* balloon. Time out here didn't feel stagnant like it did in my room. I walked and walked and tried to make sense of what the hospital stay would mean. After two full years of experiencing the uncertain tides of symptoms, the idea of receiving a concrete diagnosis felt like it might be a shoreline I could finally set foot on. A diagnosis would mean that when people asked why I had quit the cross-country team, I could give an answer other than the vague one I usually gave, "I got sick." It would mean that the voice inside my head, the one that jeered *you're faking all of this, you freak*, would finally be silenced. It would mean that I could finally, finally believe in my own body again. I could learn to trust my symptoms rather than minimizing my own pain because someone else had told me too many times it wasn't real or wasn't enough.

When my mom and I arrived at the hospital a week later, I took in a last breath of exhaust-tinged air before heading through the doors. Inside was all heels clacking against tile, the murmur of small groups talking, an impossibly high ceiling, the gravity of thousands of people tucked away in their own individual rooms, bodies vulnerable in their want for answers; the lobby felt like being in a kind of cathedral. At the front desk, I pressed my thumb down on a fingerprint reader. "Sweetheart, this way you'll be able to check in with your finger the next time you come back," a woman said. I wanted to tell her I hoped I would never return, but I thanked her instead and smiled.

My mom and I walked past the gift shop that sold overpriced candy and bracelets etched with messages like "FAITH," "HOPE," and "LOVE." Past the glass of an atrium where trees fought the building for light. Into an elevator, out. Down a hall, all the doors closed or barely cracked, into a room. The brochure had featured pictures of rooms bathed in light with views of the gothic architecture on campus, but mine was dim. Because it was a corner room, a small window gave a view of the same building I was staying in. "Make yourself comfortable," a nurse told me. I took a seat on the clean, taut sheets of the hospital bed and my mom perched where she would stay for the next three days: on a blue oversized armchair that doubled as her bed. As I lay back in bed, my body felt less like my body—something that, when the confluence of limb and blood and brain worked together just right, seemed like magic—and more like a set of numbers: a baseline heart rate, a weight, blood pressure. I found pleasure, in that moment, in my frame, which felt wiry and slim. I had whittled myself down until I was the smallest I had ever been. As a result, it felt like part of me had escaped the hospital. The nurses could take my vitals and put them on a chart for other people to read, but I could control what I consumed. No one would see that but me.

An electrode technician entered and began dotting my scalp with cold glue. I flinched, not because it hurt in any way, but because I didn't want to be there. I felt guilty immediately for thinking so; I was lucky to be there, lucky that my parents had paid, lucky that I was someone who could access answers. If I stared straight ahead, I was forced to see myself in the reflection of the "bathroom" mirror, one that was open and in the center of the room. I looked like the brochure hinted I might: an overgrown child. My hair, pieced apart for the electrode placement, looked like it had been mussed from a long nap, and a thick rainbow-colored tendril of twenty-six electrode wires cascaded from my scalp like the tail of a My Little Pony. I had the bright yellow "FALL RISK" socks the hospital gave me on my feet, oversized sweatpants from when I had run in the Outdoor

Conference meet my first year of college, and a flannel shirt from Andrea, who had let me borrow it when I realized I didn't own a button-down.

"Will you open your shirt?" the technician asked, so I did. My mom politely turned her head. The technician stared at my chest without flinching and attached cold sensors around my breasts and near my clavicle. Not wanting to see such intimate parts of my body in a setting like this one, where breasts and ribs and collarbones are reduced to placement dots on a diagram, I did not look down.

"This is your heart rate monitor," the technician told me once she had allowed me to button up. She held up a Game Boy-sized device in front of me so I could see it before she tied it loosely around my neck. "And here's your EEG monitor," she said, affixing another passport-sized pouch.

"I look like a tourist," I told my mom, but neither of us laughed. I wasn't going anywhere.

A different nurse entered the room and confirmed that my mom was my Adult Observer. She explained the plan for my stay: My mom was to keep an eye on me (which was impossible not to do, as I was literally tethered to the floor and had the option to walk about three steps to the bathroom or stay in bed), and she was to press a button if I became episodic, which would alert the doctors scanning brain waves that they should analyze mine extra carefully at that time. In addition, a camera in the center of the room, one that looked like the shiny, bulbous eye of a fly, was going to be trained on me the entire time. The wires hooked to my head and heart would communicate information about the health of my interior. The goal was to catch an episode so that doctors could officially diagnose me.

While I wanted to know what was going on with my health, I also felt an immense amount of pressure as I sat wired up in bed. I felt laid bare. I knew my parents were deeply worried and wanted answers. I knew my doctor wanted concrete evidence of something—anything. But what if the stay yielded nothing? It seemed like another way I could fail, like my body wasn't sick enough but also untrustworthy or unreadable. Or another sign that all of this was in my own head.

* * *

Before our hearts could murmur through wire, before the waves of our brains could be mapped, there was still an urge to name illness, to make meaning from mystery. In the seventh century BCE, a man was confined to his bed for observation. There, he "cried like a goat, he groaned, he shuddered, (and) he talked a lot." His body twitched and quivered, out of his control.

Contemporary Assyriologist Troels Pank Arbøll, who studied the tablet's cuneiform containing this story, noticed something that others hadn't: a mouth from which a forked tongue flickered. Following the lines, he began to discern the shape of a head adorned with a horn, a slumped belly, and two sturdy legs. The creature was a physical representation of *bennu,* a demon responsible for causing erratic motion and animal sound in previously healthy people. At the time, these symptoms were believed to be acquired "in or near a gate, (cattle) pen, river, uncultivated plot, or a corner." People could protect themselves from *bennu.* If they noticed the demon approaching, they could yell, "It is he!" and they would be spared. If they failed to guard themselves against illness, they were feared to be contagious and kept isolated in bed.

This is far from the only narrative crafted about the origins of illness, or seizure-like symptoms. In ancient Mesopotamia, people who seized were believed to have been taken by "the Hand of Sîn." In the village of Slätthög in Småland, Sweden, pouring a child's bathwater on the ground meant spirits of the underworld would seek their revenge through seizures. Being epileptic, throughout history, could mean being forced to live in an isolated room for the span of your life, being forcibly sterilized, or being forced to undergo exorcism. Most familiar to me, as I had read the story countless times while growing up, is the story in the Bible about the boy who foams at the mouth and grinds his teeth, becomes rigid and cannot speak. "You unbelieving and perverse generation," Jesus tells the crowd that has gathered around. Jesus brings the boy close to him and rebukes the demon that's been causing his symptoms; the boy walks away, completely healed. That epilepsy was associated with evil was not lost on me.

Though in some ways the mythologization of illness makes a sort of sense (we as humans want to have a way to understand ourselves and other people, and narrative can help with that), these stories seeped into public consciousness enough that policy, healthcare, and people's perception (my own included) have been shaped in a dark way. There are a few common threads that appear in these narratives and subsequent attempts to "cure" an individual. First, seizing, or seizure-like symptoms, are caused by a demon, something evil that has occupied the body of an otherwise healthy person. Second, a person who experienced seizures has historically been deemed not worthy of relationships, the ability to reproduce, access to public spaces—or even, sometimes, to live. Third, if only a person would do all they could to avoid sin and guard themselves against it, then they would stay well. This last one probably impacted me most. Family frequently told me they were praying that God would heal me, which felt complicated. On one hand, I accepted—and still accept—their prayer as a deep and beautiful form of love; they speak my name at the dinner table every night and hope for me to feel at home in my body again, which is something I hold dear. But on the other hand, when I heard that at my sickest, I felt anger. I didn't want to hope for a miracle. I wanted real answers from doctors and a way to move forward in the world without relying on divine intervention. The questions people asked me during that time and in the years that followed felt similar: Do you think you run too much? Have you paid attention to what you're eating? What about the weather? Have you tried *this* diet? Have you gone to see *this* doctor at *that* clinic? When people asked how long it had been since my last episode, and I could say something like a month or more, they expressed praise and responded, "Maybe they're gone for good."

The implication of these different questions and efforts toward care, to me as a patient, were that I wasn't doing enough to heal myself. Instead of being able to articulate that to well-wishers back then, I took my anger out on myself, on my own body for being so unruly. I wanted to be someone who drank green juice, did yoga to reduce stress, saw every specialist recommended by friends and people on the internet, ran just the right amount at a pace that wasn't too fast or slow, accepted—and received—a miracle, and became well for the rest of my life. But I wasn't. And even if I was, I still would have been sick. I knew that somewhere deep down, and I know it now. The way we talk about disability, and the way that it's been shaped throughout history, means that it's difficult to have conversations with people where I can say the episodes really aren't that bad; it's people's reactions that hurt me. As Michelle Mary Lelwica writes in *Shameful Bodies*, both able-bodied and disabled people are harmed by these stories we've been told about disability. "The belief that a better body = a normal body = an able body is difficult to question in part because dominant religious/cultural narratives constantly reinforce these equations, and in part because we regularly benefit from them," she writes. The problem is that no one can attain a perfect body and/or keep it forever; able-bodiedness is temporary for everyone, meaning that, as Lelwica writes with emphasis, "*every*body has a stake in dismantling the able-bodied/normative ideal that *no*body can achieve."

When I entered Duke University Hospital to test whether I was having seizures or not, I was still largely unaware of these cultural constructs and the fact that my shame stemmed from something larger than myself. But I did know, somewhere deep down inside, that as much as I wanted a diagnosis, I did not want *that* one. My own lack of information about epilepsy meant that I pictured a rolling back of the eyes, gnashing of tongue, and collapsing onto the ground. Even in my own sickness, my perception of disability was so skewed by cultural narratives that I stigmatized other people's experiences. I didn't want to be like them. I also resisted the idea that if I were diagnosed, the condition would last forever. At the time, I conceived of my episodes like some kind of strange animal I wanted to hunt down and kill. I thought I could eradicate my symptoms permanently if their removal was violent enough. I would smother them with pills, run long enough that they would be stamped away, cut enough weight from my frame that they would disappear.

I wonder now how many of these metaphors came from within myself and how much of my own narrative was shaped by the myths that people have used to explain illness for much of time. I wish now that I could have admitted what I was most scared of: that I would not have a normal life. I wanted to know what it was like to love and to be loved by a partner, to not fear what they might do to me if or when I was incoherent. I wanted to know that I would be able to someday find a job without hiding a part of myself that might very well break through despite my best efforts. I wanted to feel comfortable in my body again. I wanted other people to accept who I was and accept my episodes without feeling an urge to pray them away, offer me pseudoscience as a cure, or look away in shame. I wonder how much self-harm I might have saved myself had I had a gentler way of thinking about disability, about a body's vulnerabilities, about the way there is still so much beauty to be found in a form that occasionally lapses.

*   *   *

I was woken up in the middle of the first night by the machines next to me beeping. Nurses rushed in. My mom sat up in her bed, eyes puffy with lack of sleep. Someone flipped the fluorescent lights on. "Her heart rate is in the 30s," a nurse said. I sat up, irritated.

"She's an athlete," my mom said. "She runs marathons." I was too tired to correct her, to reframe her sentence in past tense. The whole thing felt like some kind of twisted metaphor: I was healthy enough that my heart rate looked like an athlete's, but I was in the hospital because I was somehow sick. It wasn't lost on me that the nurse was speaking about me in third person, as if I wasn't in the room. It felt like an echo of all the doctors who had come before, reassuring me that I was okay even when I wasn't, filling my charts with observations of whether I was or was not close to tears during each visit rather than precise descriptions of the symptoms I disclosed. The nurses left the room and we tried our best to sleep.

In the morning, everything looked dour under the harsh over-head light: linoleum streaked with wheel marks, my hair greasier than the day before, the ivory sink out of place adjacent to a wall of clunky wires and monitors. All the hovering nurses checking in on numbers, the beeping of machines, the knowledge that in some other room, the waves of my brain were taking shape without me there to see. My mom, exhausted, asked how I felt. I snapped "fine" more aggressively than I would have liked. In reality, I felt anxious *because* I felt fine. No tinge of pressure or feeling of an oncoming storm. I wanted to succumb to an episode, to feel ill when I was supposed to, and the fact that I felt good was frustrating. I was wasting money, wasting time. After a nurse took my morning numbers, a doctor rapped at the door. I sat up straight in my bed, smoothed down my flannel, and tried to look as appropriate as I could, given the circumstances. My mom stood from her chair. It wasn't just the doctor who came in, but about six other people, all of them wearing white coats and carrying clipboards.

"Ms. Alnes," the doctor said as a way of introduction. "Are you comfortable with the residents-in-training observing this?" Wanting to be good, I nodded my head yes. Really, I wanted the doctor alone. I wanted to take down my wall of feigned calm and tell him that I was both frantic for answers and terrified by the prospect of them. I wanted to cry. Some of the residents looked not much older than me, and I had the urge to tell them, *I wear normal clothes in my real life! I have friends! I am in college!* I wanted to show them something I'd written or my transcript or a list of times from past cross-country meets, something that would prove that I had a life outside this three-foot radius.

So much of being a patient is experiencing a distillation of the self into characteristics someone else deems to be the most important. My first intake form at the neurologist's office freshman year, for example, describes me as: "a Freshman at Elon University. Her parents live in Tulsa, OK. She denies alcohol, tobacco use, or sexual activity. She is a Freshman on the Women's Cross-Country team." The doctor knew about my past "left great toe surgery," my great-grandmother's stroke, and my seasonal allergies, but not about how lonely it felt to be a thousand miles away from my family with a coach who pressured me to keep running. He didn't know about my love of language, both as a writer and a reader, and how hearing the videos of my voice echo broken sentences back pierced me with an acute kind of sadness. At the neurologist's office, the collapse in my dorm room turned into an "episode of syncope," and down the road, my repeated speech issues would be labeled "aphasia." To be a patient, at times, is to feel dislocated from your own sense of self, to see your experience translated into a language that is impenetrable, no matter how closely you try to listen.

Being a patient also means playing a game of appearances, one I had an advantage in already as a white, thin woman. I knew not to cry too much, not to inflect very much emotion when describing my symptoms. I knew to dress well enough to convey good mental health. So when the head neurologist, surrounded by his residents, asked how I was feeling, I said, "Fine." I explained that I was experiencing none of the usual pre-episode symptoms and that I felt remarkably clear-headed. The residents scribbled notes. The doctor explained that throughout the day, nurses would be coming in and out to do a series of tests that they hoped might help induce an episode, and I was instructed to stay awake into the night as long as I could in order to stress my body through exhaustion. The doctor asked if there might be anything else I could do to mirror triggers in the outside world, and my mom asked if there was a way I could exercise; the doctor said a stationary bike with no resistance would be wheeled in shortly. The doctor let us know that my brain waves looked normal so far (*an unremarkable brain*, I joked to myself, mimicking the medical terms I'd seen for years on my charts) and that he would be back the next morning to provide another update. We thanked him, and the whole group shuffled out, ready to bear witness to their next case study.

* * *

During the period that Essie Honiball probably should have been hospitalized, she reflected that an unlikely source—the stringent rules of Cornelius's experiment—gave her courage to keep going. When I think about Essie during this time—unable to climb stairs, her ears ringing with pain, experiencing full-body cramps that rendered her too rigid to move—it seems, from the outside, that eating just three pieces of fruit per day would add to her pain, not offer relief. But, as she writes, "This meant progress and gave me courage for what lay ahead. The miracle of the diet was, however, that I could indeed keep going and I was making progress."

In the hospital, I better understood the comfort Essie took in withholding most foods from herself. I was allowed to eat whatever I wanted during my stay, but I had a visceral fear of eating the hospital meals, which loomed in my imagination as being exceptionally dense, congealed, and full of fatty calories. Before the test, I had asked my mom to stop at Whole Foods, where we had picked up pounds of pre-steamed sweet potatoes, fruit, and bags of popcorn. My fears around food at the time precipitated a moodiness that engulfed me more often than not. I got irritated with my mom when she encouraged me to buy something like a protein bar, and I was so swept up in calculating *what was healthy, what would keep me thin, what would stave off hunger,* or *what would happen if I let myself eat a bite of something I wasn't supposed to,* that I can imagine I wasn't very much fun to be around.

Though I didn't talk about my eating habits with any level of transparency at the time (to speak about my fears would force me to engage with them in an intellectual way, and I just wanted to *feel* the fear of fat, not consider the potential pitfalls of demonizing an entire category of food out loud), I think my mom understood that something was going on. In the morning, after the doctor left, she offered to get me a coffee from the lobby and returned with a drink and a surprise: She pulled a sleeve of Peeps, my favorite, from behind her back. I opened the packet and bit off the soft, sugar-coated head of a yellow chick, consoling myself with the fact that they were high in carbs and low in fat. Even if my methods weren't as pure as three pieces of fruit a day, controlling what I ate while sitting in my hospital bed made me feel that I had power. I metered out my rations of fruit and steamed potatoes, asking myself with each bite if I had earned it. The answer was always no, but my hunger got the best of me.

*   *   *

The days in the hospital passed like a held breath. We waited for answers. Each night became a comedy routine of sorts when my mom and I were woken up by nurses who were deeply concerned about my low heart rate. (It seemed especially ironic to me that my comparable vitals from my entire stay had been written up on a whiteboard in the room, and still we had to convince whoever was tending to me that I was, in fact, okay.) The neurologist and his team visited me each morning— as I progressively grew greasier and more restless—to inform us that nothing of note had appeared on my brain waves. My mom and I watched shows about house renovations, housewives shrieking at one another, and toddlers competing in pageants. We took turns moving our legs on the resistance-less stationary bike. We ate popcorn out of red Solo cups, trying to stay awake late into the night despite our boredom.

Throughout the day, technicians came by to conduct tests. I was asked to blow repeatedly for two minutes straight for the hyperventilation test, which left me lightheaded but episode-less. I stared at flashing lights with no result. With each test that produced no change in my brain waves, I felt more and more frustrated. It seemed like I existed in a state where I was sick enough that parts of my life were interrupted, but not sick enough for my condition to be real. In that space, I felt the familiar anger of failure rising in me. Why had I not been able to attend all my classes if nothing was wrong with me? Why did I collapse into incoherence in Peru? Was this how my whole life was going to be, a gingerly dance between my own experience in my body and what the doctors told me? The fear that ate at me most was the potential that all of this was in my head, that somehow I had lost my grip on reality.

On the final morning, the doctor and his group of residents entered. "How are you feeling?" the doctor asked.

"Honestly, just fine," I told him. "I don't feel any sort of hint that an episode is coming."

The doctor nodded and took a note. "This happens more often than you think. Patients come in for long spans of time without experiencing an event."

"It's frustrating," I said, and he nodded in agreement.

The neurologist said, despite the absence of a full-blown episode, they'd noted "neuronal dysfunction in the posterior right temporal region" of my brain, the region that controls language production. The two sides of my brain moved at slightly different speeds, creating a potential platform for migraines or seizures. Though it was useful information in some ways, the visit produced no conclusive answers. My mom asked questions about what would come next. I was allowed to stop taking my seizure medication, if I wished, and monitor my symptoms under the care of a neurologist as the months went on. If ever my episodes became more frequent and interfered with the quality of my life, I could check myself in for another continuous EEG to try to pin down exactly what the issue was. The residents took their notes.

When it was time for me to be discharged, a technician and nurse entered the room. The nurse asked if I would consent to have my picture taken with her; she was giving a presentation the following month at a conference and a visual would be helpful. Before considering where the photo might go or what people might take from it, I said yes. I smoothed down my hospital sheets, straightened my sweatpants, and tried to sit up as straight as I could in bed. The nurse made a show of standing at my bedside, gingerly pinching one of my electrodes between her fingertips. The technician took a series of photos while I tried to guess at whether I was supposed to look happy, serious, or sad. I didn't have the words to articulate how I felt in that moment, being discharged without a real diagnosis—shame that my body withheld answers, rage that I was starting my third year undiagnosed, immense fear that I would continue to live with the possibility of my legs collapsing, mouth slurring words, or memory lapsing at any minute. When the technician scrolled through the digitals to get my approval, my eyes looked vaguely empty and my mouth was set in an attempt at a smile. With wires unspooling from my scalp, wires infiltrating my clothing, and monitors in the background, I looked like the star of an infomercial. While I am very grateful for the work that doctors do, I was in such a sour mood at the time that I imagined my picture being used as a testament to *the power of finding answers for patients! Giving them hope!* The technician undid the rest of my electrodes, and I tried not to look as deflated as I felt. To keep myself from crying, I daydreamed about a long run down the centerline of the farmland roads.

CHAPTER 14

Pints of Milk and Boiled Potatoes (Fruit Yourself! Root Yourself!)

BY THE TIME SUMMER ROLLED AROUND, THERE WERE MANY ways that my life, at least from the outside, looked like the perfect ending to a Testify! post on 30BaD. My episodes had not returned after my stay in the hospital, and I remained unmedicated. I was still following a stringent eating plan, in which I had eliminated most sugar and fat. My limbs were slim enough that a friend's mom told me my arms looked as thin as bird bones; I took it as a compliment rather than an expression of concern. After walking for much of the spring, I had started running again, a return to the way of moving through the world I loved most. I could have put a slideshow set to an electronic beat on YouTube of me waterskiing at the lake! Lounging on a floatie with a slice of summer watermelon in hand! Flipping a tire at the track, my biceps as shredded as they've ever been!

But inside, the dream of finding THE ANSWER had soured like the juice of rotten fruit forgotten in a refrigerator drawer. I had believed so fervently that if I just got my episodes under control, that if I just wrangled my body into submission, I would be happy. And I felt anything but. I had three months until senior year started, which meant the end of college was on the horizon, and I had no idea what I was supposed to do with the rest of my life. Would I be bedridden in six months or remain clear-headed? When I had dared to hope at the finish line of the marathon, the symptoms had come crashing back in. They obliterated my tepid attempts to rebuild my life. It seemed like no matter how good I tried to be, how pure, how fanatical about my sleep habits and stress and the records I kept, these episodes would shape my life in ways that were out of my control. In some ways, that summer felt like an extension of my hospital stay, like I was tethered to one spot, under strict observation. I had once become episodic while in the lake, so that summer, I wasn't allowed to swim without someone else around. I had to ask my little brother for rides and leave my mom Post-it Notes listing the time I left for runs so she could come look for me if I was gone too long. My family frequently asked how I was feeling. The gestures were loving, but I felt smothered. I felt stretched between a desire to be twenty and free, flaunting a figure I'd sacrificed too many nights of communal meals or spontaneous outings for, and the knowledge that I had to, for my own safety, allow myself to be cared for in the ways that my family offered. Rather than turn my anger outward, I directed it where I always had—at my own body.

Illness too often reduced the scope of my focus to my own perceptions of the world: How did I feel at any given moment? Was the pressure in my head just normal morning grogginess, or would the day go south? Was skipping my daily run a product of fear, normal summer relaxation, or a sign that I felt the aura of something bad about to happen? Because I had not been intimate physically with anyone, not enough to see their flaws or weird human habits, and because I had been stuck in an apartment for the past semester watching curated videos of Freelee with her six-pack and slender hips, I had a skewed vision of what desire might look like, and what it might mean to love a body for what it really was.

My summer job cut through those illusions. Based on a neighbor's recommendation, a couple hired me to work for their bed-and-breakfast, which catered especially toward Christian couples on their honeymoons. My mom drove me to work most mornings, where I helped with breakfast prep (usually making sure a casserole didn't get burned, a task I failed at more than once), as well as serving guests juice and coffee. While the guests were eating, my boss would coax me out from behind the counter and tell me to go socialize. (Trust me, I knew enough at the time to recognize that the *last* thing a honeymooning couple probably wants is a random twenty-year-old with no talent for small talk hovering near the edge of their table in the morning—or anytime, really.) With my boss watching, I would bring a pitcher of ice water to each table and make sure to ask if they had enjoyed the lake or the nearby amusement park. Up close, the couples always appeared fresh-faced. They wore outfits that had clearly been selected to show their unity as a pair: sets of navy and khaki, cherry red and denim. They were polite, their voices hushed. I was envious of their lives; they had found someone who loved them. They were on their honeymoon. The closest I had come to letting myself want in the past couple years had been with Ben, and even that was the furthest possible brush with romance.

It was only later, when the guests had rolled down the gravel drive and I took up my cleaning duties, that I got a more realistic view of love. Unlike the pressed and polite versions of themselves in the lobby, the rooms were strewn with detritus that punctured any vision of perfection. There were empty pimple cream tubes in the trash, hairs plastered to the glass wall of the shower and coiled on the tile, wet towels on the ground, pill bottles peeking out from toiletry bags, sheets (my beautiful, taut, triple-sheeted beds, always inspected by my former-military boss) rumpled and undone, a bottle of pop half-finished beside the bed, hair growth cream, the serrated edge of a condom wrapper on the carpeted floor, jets of the Jacuzzi releasing dirt when I checked whether or not they had been used, a lingerie set with tags still attached hanging in the closet. My bosses included one album in each room—Kenny Rogers's "Love Songs"—and my favorite cleaning task was to see whether or not the CD was in or out of the small boom box next to each bed, a sign that it had been used the night before.

The rooms gave me reassurance I hadn't found in other spaces. Everyone, as evidenced through their tinctures and creams, those empty tubes riddled with promise, had insecurities. Everyone was different in their private life than in public. Everyone was deeply human. And they had all found someone to share the cramped space of a hotel bathroom with, someone to love. These were things that I probably knew on some level before, but surveying dozens and dozens of rooms, in all their gross glory, made me feel so much less alone.

* * *

From the outside, Freelee and Durianrider's life together seemed perfect: two wildly in shape people in love, cycling hundreds of miles side by side, saving the animals and the planet through their ethical diet. They ate bananas on tropical beaches together. Freelee made necklaces from dried oranges. They embraced the power of raw fruit and shared how being vegan had helped them lose weight, stay fit, get six-packs, clear up their candida, and live how humans were *intended* to live.

The reality the couple communicated via social media was one that I, at the time, internalized as being the full truth. That's the beauty—and danger—of a parasocial relationship; you start to think you know a person based on their posts, when all you're really seeing is a set of curated snippets. There's a chance that the truth I had interpreted was, in fact, a sort of truth; Freelee and Durianrider's lives, at the time, might have included an abundance of raw fruit, healthfulness, and love for each other. But as honest as we are on social media, and as much as we share, it's never a vessel that can communicate the fullness of our real lives. Reality is often more nuanced than the glossy, stagnant façade of social media. In Freelee and Durianrider's case, at some point in the years after creating 30BaD, they had begun experimenting off-camera with introducing cooked food into their diet.

Because of the sheer quantity of material the couple distributed daily on platforms from 30BaD to YouTube to Instagram, it is possible that I missed an announcement related to their diet pivot. And, because Freelee and Durianrider did not respond to interview requests in which I asked about when, how, and why they elected to incorporate cooked food into their diet, I want to be clear that, in this section, I am working from my own memory, posts archived by the Wayback Machine, interviews published online, and YouTube videos that Freelee and Durianrider posted during this time period.

On June 5, 2012, in a video posted to Freelee's YouTube channel titled "How to start a RAW FOOD / Raw till 4 Diet today!" Freelee lays out her steps for success:

Step one: "Educate yourself and get excited!!" (Cue video of Freelee dancing in a bikini in the shower, dark hair flailing to the rhythm, a voiceover of Freelee saying, "I knew I'd found the holy grail.")

Step two: "Join our community at 30Bananasaday.com . . . And also subscribe to myself and Durianrider's blogs and Facebook updates for more tips."

Step three: Find a buddy. There's a montage of Freelee on her back, being lifted into the air by a friend's feet (like a child doing an airplane upside down), and in between shots we see a photo of a pear and strawberry with worried faces running from a leering banana with an unpeeled lower half. Over this, Freelee is telling listeners that they can eat two fruit meals and then end their day with a "high carb, cooked vegan meal at night."

At the time, I remember watching this video in my apartment and feeling a sense of disbelief wash over me. I wasn't at all upset that the pair had incorporated a wider variety of foods into their diet—they were and are entitled to eat however they feel is best for their bodies— but as someone who had begun to believe in the rhetoric offered to me time and time again in different videos and posts, I had my own questions: Didn't cooked food pollute the body? Weren't steamed potatoes a toxin? I had watched videos like Durianrider's 2009 "RAW FOOD VEGAN FALLS OFF THE COOKED FOOD WAGON" in which he puts ripe, raw tomatoes into the microwave and jokes, "Where's the fruit button? I'm not gonna get enough lycopene if I eat them that fresh." Finding the microwave too difficult to work, he ends his skit by caving and eating the tomatoes raw. He blamed our reliance on cooked food on "a bunch of idealists writing books and selling cooked food instruments like microwaves and ovens, trying to make money." I remember reading "Freelee the Fruitionist's" posts denigrating cooked food, like, "How do i [sic] know im [sic] not eating enough calories from fruit?": "Cooked food starts to look and smell good," "Cooked food looks more then [sic] the toxic, second rate slop it really is," and "Your [sic] actually eating cooked food and reading this." I remember watching, in November 2011, when Freelee posted an eleven-minute video explaining how to "get rid of cooked food cravings." In that video, she emphasized that eating enough fruit could help anyone who was tempted by rice, pasta, or potatoes. And yet, here Freelee was, suddenly promoting eating steamed potatoes as a positive thing?

Later in the Raw Till 4 introduction video posted in 2012, with no context about why, how, or when she made the change, Freelee loads up a box with quarts of organic orange juice, saying, "Myself, I even have pasteurized juice now and don't have a problem with it." (She had previously only permitted herself to drink freshly squeezed orange juice that she made at home.) She then tells viewers to stock up on ten pounds or more of organic potatoes so that they are readily available at home, or whatever root vegetables suit their fancy ("Note: Steamed is healthiest" she posts, with no explanation as to why she believes this cooking method is healthiest). She jokes that ten pounds might not even be enough; people should have as many potatoes around as possible so they aren't tempted by meat, cheese, or even computer keyboards if they get hungry enough. In this video, Freelee emphasizes that these cooked food options are "nowhere near as good as fruit, but they're awesome at this stage in your journey." From the language in the video, it seems to me that Freelee was offering cooked food as an option for people who might have a hard time shifting from a standard diet to raw veganism.

But about a year or so after posting this footage, Freelee and Durianrider began promoting Raw Till 4 as a sort of sister diet to 30 Bananas a Day. In Freelee's *Raw Till 4 Diet* e-book, she writes that her mom, who "adopted a partly raw lifestyle" saw "great results" and inspired the creation of RT4. The rules of Raw Till 4 were pretty simple: eat raw until 4 p.m., at which time "potatoes, root veggies, rice, gluten-free pasta," pasta sauce, broccoli, spinach, salad, and really, anything "high-carb" with less than 1,000 mg of salt and less than 10% fat permitted.

While Freelee and Durianrider were promoting Raw Till 4, they also kept their 30BaD website going. There, the rules stayed the same: no cooked food, no pasteurized juice, no sugar added to smoothies. This, at the time, confused me: Did they believe in the rules on the 30BaD site or had they just neglected to take the page down? Why did they post new comments on raw forums there if they believed that cooked food was now okay? What did it mean that both diets were viable options? Was one better than another?

Enough people had questions about the couple's pivot from an all-raw diet to one that included cooked food that Durianrider participated in an interview published to fruit-powered.com in December 2013. When asked if there was "a specific event or was there a realization over time . . . to expand the focus of your lifestyle promotions to include cooked carbohydrates?" Durianrider responded, "The raw food movement has pretty much died . . . We just want to end the purity mindset and help people make better dietary and lifestyle choices instead of trying to get them to go full throttle into something only a very small percentage of the planet can actually do due to finances and situational convenience." He continued, "We have done the math and seen that people do raw foods for just a few weeks and that's it . . . We push fruit as much if not more than ever."

When asked if they had shifted from a wholly raw approach to including cooked food or if it was just a backup, Durianrider commented, "We are very hardline on our forum, 30BaD. We want to give people that absolute pure raw experience so they can work out what direction they want to head [in] . . . They can stay with that or add in other high-carb vegan foods. It's up to them. Depends on their goals and current situation."

Durianrider, in the interview, commented that, from his perspective, the shift to posting about their inclusion of cooked foods led to "Off-the-charts subscribers on all social media outlets. For December 2013, I will get over 3.4 million views alone on my main channel." I was one of those viewers, peering in to look at a community I was realizing more and more that I had never truly been a part of. What the diet had given me was a certainty that I had otherwise been lacking, a framework through which to see illness and justify my disdain for my own body. When the rules changed, for me it was as if the mirage of it all suddenly dissipated. If Freelee and Durianrider could change the foundation of their system overnight, then what was I believing in?

*   *   *

Perhaps what was more alluring than the details of any diet's rules, at least for me, was just the presence of structure, the idea that there was something in the world that remained simple, straightforward, and unwavering. At the time, it was easier for me to believe that something was wrong with me—I lacked willpower, I wasn't brave enough to try—than to consider the idea that maybe there were other people out there who tried to give off the illusion that they had their lives under control, while in reality, the truth was more complex—and subsequently more relatable. When I look back at fruit-eaters through history, this idea that we sometimes resist sharing publicly the messy parts of ourselves becomes clearer. Arnold Ehret, who wrote about how fruit and fasting cured him of a heart condition, claimed to thrive for a time on mandarin oranges while disclosing in his autobiography that he actually enjoyed cake every single day. (The cake he ate sounds amazing: "Turkish barley, first roasted a little and then shredded, some brown almonds and burned sugar. Over the whole a crust of sweet icing is poured.") Ehret does not mention his sweet tooth in his diet book, in which he tells readers to stick to fresh fruit, raw celery, lettuce, carrots, and beets in order to keep their bodies mucus-free. Basil Shackleton, the man who swore he had a bilharzia bug wreaking "utter destruction!" on his kidneys, turned to wine, spirits, and cigarettes every few months before getting back on the grape wagon. Essie Honiball once got a craving for milk after nearly a decade of abstaining. She stopped at a little cafe, bought a two-liter milk carton, and drank the entire thing. "And she felt wonderful," Anoeschka, Essie's biographer, told me. "Super super guilty, but it was soothing to her stomach. The whole day, at intervals, she would stop and buy more milk, and more milk. She drank and she drank and she drank liters of milk that day and she felt so much better." After a day or two, Anoeschka can't remember now, Essie went back to eating fruit and put the incident behind her.

I wonder now how different Essie's life might have been had she used the milk incident as a means of connecting with other people rather than as an example with which to set herself apart. Her forays into eating cooked food and chugging milk hardened her resolve to continue eating fruit exclusively. What would have happened if she had softened, even slightly, instead? Might she have been able to partake in a biscuit at a friend's house every now and then? Or a cup of tea, even if more for the warmth of community than the actual beverage itself? Instead, not confessing to anyone in her day-to-day life that she had succumbed to temptation, she stayed on her isolated path. Around town, she began to hear things like, "Oh, you probably don't mind that we no longer invite you to dinner, but you are no longer one of us." Essie felt like an outcast and began to experience adverse health effects as a result. She writes in her memoir that she experienced nightmares followed by "psychosomatic symptoms" like "troublesome pains and sensations," even though all of her medical examinations showed she was in "excellent health." Anoeschka described the symptoms that she had witnessed as "convulsions or hiccups."

In 1973, Essie was saved from loneliness by her second husband, T. O. Honiball, a famous South African cartoonist. She, in turn, saved him from poor health by secretly converting him to fruitarianism. She lists out the sly way in which she transitioned a man who loved "meat, fish, rice and gravy, chocolate cake, ice cream, curry and rice," to a man who sat down at the dinner table and said, "For goodness' sake, rather go and fetch my fruit." She started off by simplifying his diet (phase one) and offering him "the finest fruit" she could find. To fulfill phase two, "Farewell to all products from the animal kingdom," she feigned forgetting to put the milk in the fridge so that it soured and offered him fruit pulp instead. Phase three was perhaps her boldest: "Farewell to the stove," and phase four signified a full conversion to fruit, "supplemented with what may be found necessary through more research in the future." Essie says that when T. O. finally realized he had been converted, "his excess mass, his headaches and even ugly moles on his back slowly but surely started disappearing and that he could again climb stairs without stopping half way to pant for breath."

*   *   *

It was the black-and-white mentality that had drawn me to the 30BaD community in the first place, the way that Freelee and Durianrider could order the world into good and evil, fruit and bags of blood. After they shifted to cooked food after 4:00 p.m., it wasn't that I suddenly lost hope in the diet itself (I was eating Peeps in a hospital, after all), it was something deeper. If they could move the goalposts on the very foundation of their beliefs—and in a way that seemed so arbitrary to me (what changed in the human body after 4 p.m. that made cooked food okay?)—then what else wasn't true about what they said? Maybe it wasn't even the pair recanting their rules that really broke me, but what I saw as hypocrisy. How was it okay to sell e-books about going raw and keep a raw food forum going without editing the rules while also claiming that cooked potatoes and pasta were healthy?

I wasn't the only one who took issue with the changes in Freelee and Durianrider's direction. In 2011, 2012, and 2013, Durianrider had enjoyed attending the Woodstock Fruit Festival, and Freelee had attended in 2012 and 2013. The festival is probably exactly what you think based on the name. A bunch of fruitarians head to Camp Walden, in the Adirondacks, New York, every summer to eat from a buffet of endless fruit, dive into lakes, participate in massage trains, do pull-ups on trees, hula hoop, show each other silly bike tricks, do yoga, juggle oranges, and let their bodies careen in acrobatic feats across wide grassy lawns. Freelee and Durianrider, alongside founder Michael Arnstein, fellow YouTubers like FullyRaw Kristina (Kristina Carrillo-Bucaram), and none other than Douglas Graham, had been "Pioneers" of Woodstock—which means they were compensated for their attendance at the festival, got a chance to speak or offer some form of a session and, for a weekend, were generally lauded as rockstars of the fruit world by people who knew them from social media. However, in November 2013, Freelee and Durianrider were "removed as Pioneers." The board of governors (including Graham) explained in a post, "Sometime in the

"Where do we start?" Freelee asks. She purses her lips.

"Where do we start?" Durianrider echoes.

They tell viewers that they had a "really good time" at the "fucking awesome event" the year before. They wish they could go back to Woodstock. But they can't, and to help them stay on track, they have a bullet-point list of reasons why.

"We got voted off," Freelee says, in a tone that reminds me of confessional footage on a show like *Survivor*, "by people who said they were friends."

"I got a call from Mike [Arnstein] a few weeks ago," Durianrider says, "and Mike was saying, you know, Harley, you got no fucking friends, they all fucking hate you, they want you out. You've been making all these backup plan videos, you've gotta take them down, and you've gotta write to such-and-such and explain that you're sorry. You've gotta fucking basically brownnose your 'friends' and let them know why you should be coming to the festival still."

While it is difficult for me to imagine a grown person calling up another grown person to say, "You've got no fucking friends, they all hate you," the impact this decision had on Freelee and Durianrider is clear. To highlight their former Board members' hypocrisy, in the video, Freelee talks about how FullyRaw Kristina's "focus is way off. It's not about the planet, the animals, and the people."

"It's about me," Durianrider concludes.

They talk about how Douglas Graham had preached in the past that 80/10/10 was not intended to be an elitist diet, inaccessible to the masses, but then later said that "raw is law." "It creates a real niche microeconomy where people feel like failures because they have a bowl of steamed rice and broccoli," Durianrider says. "Come on. You've gotta give people a backup plan. We don't live in the jungle. We live in the world of 7-Eleven." Freelee and Durianrider felt the irony of the group's split (and subsequent infinity mirror of sparring YouTube "reaction" videos) in a way that I sometimes do, too. For a community that prioritizes nonviolence and peace between different beings, both animal and human, there certainly was a lot of infighting. And over what? Some boiled potatoes. As much as Freelee and Durianrider seemed to resent the way they had been treated, in my mind, examples exist of them perpetuating similar kinds of exclusion.

An example of this is their treatment of an Israeli influencer, Henya Von Perez, who went under the moniker "Henya Mania." Henya started out on the Raw Till 4 diet in the hopes of curing herself from a chronic case of candida. She subsequently posted to Instagram that she felt "fucking awesome." She posted that meeting Freelee, someone she credited for getting her into social media and YouTube, was like a "long lost vegan sista." Henya remained a high-carb, raw vegan for about a year before confessing in a video that she had given up that lifestyle. "I've been Fully Raw, Raw Till 4, Starch Solution, Banana Island, all those things. I've done them and to be completely honest with you guys, I did not feel good on them," she says. Henya makes it clear, in her video, that her opening up about how Raw Till 4 and the other diets didn't work for her was not meant to be a personal attack on Freelee and Durianrider. Instead, she called for the vegan community to come together, to stop the infighting, and to focus on what mattered: the animals. "You can also be vegan by just being a vegan," she says. "It doesn't have to be low-sodium, low-fat, this and that, blah blah blah. It does not have to be that way in order for you to be vegan." In a Facebook post, she re-emphasized her point, writing, "I've always promoted eating whatever you wanna eat so long as it's vegan, be it 10 banana smoothies or hummus and bread . . . The animals on the way to slaughter couldn't care less about your [macronutrient] ratios and they don't give a fuck what 'kind' of vegan you are."

It seems, from their videos about the matter, that Durianrider and Freelee took the evolution of Henya's eating habits as a personal sleight. "You call yourself an activist?" Durianrider says in a response video. He's sitting in the dark, only the light from his laptop illuminating his face, wearing his classic "VEGAN" T-shirt. "You've got a tattoo that says 'Animal Liberation'? No, no, no. It should be called 'Animal Commodification: How I Make Money Off My Vegan Friends.' You know what I mean?" People in the comments responded with mixed reviews. Some people wrote things like, "This video is complete destruction! Backstabbers need to be called out!" but others urged Durianrider to "stop the hate, we're all in for the same cause which is stopping the killings of our precious earthling friends! we're supposed to be a loving community."

And Durianrider's video spurred other followers to weigh in. In one, a user named LITWAI intersperses clips of Henya's YouTube videos with his own commentary. He holds his camera up just above his head and stands in what looks to be a doorway to rant. "It's obvious that she was just too fucking lazy or it was too fucking hard for her. Don't blame the lifestyle like it's not the best fucking diet out there, okay? High carb is the way to eat, okay? There's only one path for me when it comes to macronutrient ratios, and it's high carb." He speaks in a monotone voice, and his "okays" hold an edge. "If you want to be a sedentary vegan and you don't want to be an activist, then, sure, eat high-fat foods and watch Netflix all day, whatever floats your fucking boat. But you know what Harley and Freelee are trying to build? They're trying to build a community of fucking carbed-up vegans that are getting shit done and that have high energy to do it. If it is about the animals, then we're trying to create the best vegan activists that we can."

I include an excerpt from this video not because this user is exceptional, but because this type of response video, where one vegan takes another vegan down with "receipts" from their own posted YouTube video, was banal at the time. There are hundreds of response videos for any number of dramas that took place within the vegan community—covering everything from steroid use, to "gotcha" moments of vegans eating meat, to beef between influencers, to money woes, to squabbles over diet. You name it, there's probably a series of YouTube videos for it. To me, LITWAI's response feels charged with something like betrayal and feels symbolic of the pitfalls of maintaining an all-or-nothing approach to eating. If someone expressed publicly that they were living their life happily, without rules, then what did that mean for everyone else who still trusted in a plan?

The group, formerly a small set of people sharing simple gifts around a picnic table at a farm, was becoming contentious. Suddenly, spreading the vegan message on YouTube seemed to me to become a situation where one wrong word or phrase could get you castigated by the leaders of the movement in a video of their own.

*   *   *

If the goal was truly influencing people toward a vegan lifestyle, Freelee and Durianrider's raw money-making notwithstanding, then what was the problem with that? There seemed to be bigger issues at stake, like the fact that the 80/10/10 nutrition plan was created by a chiropractor who at one point had his license suspended. I'm less interested in the drama of YouTube and more invested in what these situations can teach us about intersections between profit, personal responsibility, and wellness culture. For example, is it ethical that Freelee and Durianrider continued facilitating and presumably profiting from a forum where a "hardline" version of eating was promoted when they simultaneously made public claims that a different diet worked just as well? What do we expect of an individual sharing the benefits of a way of life that works for them, and what happens when that personal belief becomes more of a public movement? Do the levels of personal responsibility—on behalf of both the leader and the potential follower—change as a result? What role should platforms like YouTube and Instagram have to protect vulnerable populations from receiving information from ˌline who give advice about nutrition and exercise?

I'm also interested in the way Woodstock's rejection of Freelee and Durianrider facilitated the kind of extremist approach to eating that led so many people to feel stuck and ashamed of their perceived failings in the first place. If the public message sent to followers of raw veganism was that cooked food was unacceptable, it didn't allow for people to have conversations about different styles of eating that might work best in their personal lives, and it didn't allow for people to share tips and tricks for remaining a high-carb, raw vegan even when fresh tropical fruit wasn't accessible or affordable to them. Instead, it brought further shame on followers who couldn't remain fully raw, for whatever reason, and set a precedent that publicly decrying someone else's diet was all right. It wasn't solely a philosophical conversation about ethics; these videos had real-life consequences. An example is a post by a 30BaD user titled, "Something feels wrong. Too wrong. Need some advice. Please!" Their post, written after Freelee and Durianrider had introduced Raw Till 4 on their other public platforms, says that they've been high-carb vegan for one year but admit "not 100%." Because they reside in a cold climate ("No, it's not an excuse!"), the fruit consists of "frost-bitten bananas, apples full of chemicals [can feel by the taste], the same with pears, moldy pineapples." Despite carbohydrates making up "85% or more" of their diet, they feel "drugged," spaced out, and weak. A B12 shot had improved their insomnia, poor concentration, and light-headedness, but at the time of posting they still felt unwell, complaining of a stuffy nose, swollen lymph nodes and dark circles under their eyes. Some of the responses to the post include:

"How many calories a day do you eat? Sounds like you need more carbs."

"I ate a cooked meal a couple weeks ago and I got those same symptoms you are describing. I wish I could give you some advice on

how to get good fruit. the only thing i can think of is move somewhere nicer :p"

"Is it possible that you have the flu? Do you have any fever? I would
find an [sic] holistic doctor to run some tests—not all doctors will
tell you to eat meat, mine doesn't. If there are deficiencies there,
you can address them from a vegan angle."

"try eating an avocado!"

To me, the comments are interesting because they offer a glimpse of
the diet's rhetoric reflected through other voices, and signal how much
people within the community believed they knew about nutrition
and health, in that they felt comfortable dispensing advice. I wonder
how many people listened to comments rather than signs their bodies
might have been giving them, and what it might have been like to have
someone give them permission to eat whatever they wanted.

What makes me most sad about all of it, in a way, is that Essie
Honiball, Arnold Ehret, and Basil Shackleton all lived lives full of
mistakes and cravings and a changing attitude toward the way they
nourished themselves, but they were too committed to the ideal of
perfection, too entranced with the way they had moralized food, to
ever admit it in a real, vulnerable way to anyone else. Instead, they tried
again and again—through memoir, through a "Scientific Method of
Eating Your Way to Health," through "before and after" photographic
evidence, through social media posts, rule books, forums, and YouTube
videos—to present fruitarianism as the natural, right way to live. In
this way, a diet that was supposed to be Eden-esque, an escape from the
pressures of society, was actually just a thorny maze with ever-changing
rules and hypocritical leaders.

Unlike the Garden of Eden, real gardens—and real narratives—
aren't as simple as Genesis presents them to be. Real gardens are full of

tangled vines, branches that have broken under the weight of what they bear, fruitless stalks, leaves browning from weather or pests, ripe flesh torn open by beak or claw. Real lives—real people—are impossible to contain in black-and-white boxes. They grow in unexpected directions. They shed what does not serve them and reach toward the things that bring them nourishment. They evolve.

CHAPTER 15

The Serpent Tricked Me

THE SPELL OF FREELEE AND DURIANRIDER WAS BROKEN FOR me when they pivoted to cooked food, but also by circumstances in my own life. When I had believed in them most, I was alone in my apartment, praying to the light of my laptop for an answer. But over the summer, at home, I couldn't spend hours letting myself be lulled by the familiar beat of "Raw (raw raw raw), Fit (fit fit fit), Bitch (bitch bitch bitch)" or watching "What I Eat In a Day" videos from a rising crop of fruit-fluencers. Instead, I paid attention to the thousands of small white flowers that clustered together on a head of Queen Anne's lace, the butterflies that flew to the lake's edge to probe for water, and the way my legs grew capable of carrying me up the steep, rocky hill that led home after I went for a run or walk each day. I snuck marshmallows from the pantry at lunch with my brother and ate ice cream with him at night when we watched the Olympics. I dove into a research project about Willa Cather, guided by my professor Dr. Schwind, and started believing in myself as a thinker again.

By the time I went back to school for the fall semester of senior year, something in me had shifted. No longer was I tempted to park my car somewhere alone so I could eat half a cake in one sitting, nor was I abstaining from meals with roommates, sure that I was superior for my ability to avoid fat. I just was. The more I lived in the world, away from my screen, the quieter the voices saying eggs were chicken "menses" and dairy was an animal "secretion" grew. I went out for froyo on a regular basis (enough that Eliza, Andrea, and I would dress exclusively in monochromatic clothing as a ritual), ate sweet potato fries for lunch, and ran because I wanted to, however far I wanted to go. I didn't consume too many of Freelee and Durianrider's videos, instead only allowing high-carb, raw vegan content into my life through a small trickle of accounts I followed on Instagram and Snapchat, where I watched women around my age eat mangoes, bike, or flaunt their fruit bodies at the beach. I spoke up in class, applied for MFA writing programs in secret, went to my first college parties, wrote bad poems, climbed a magnolia tree at dusk, and made enough new friends to realize that my own pain had shielded me from the idea that people bore the weight of their own difficult histories in their own private way.

The day before graduation, I slipped out the front door of my apartment early enough that the farmland roads were hazy with fog, like a scene in a movie from a different time. I acknowledged the details that held meaning for me: the cows with their wide eyes, the star house, the *It's a girl!* baby who had been born the year before, the still surface of a pond I always longed to disrupt, the cabin with the gnomes clustered out front like a great choir. In the past, I had knelt beside the bodies of squirrels, their intestines coiled like a bracelet of ruby-colored pearls, or an opossum with a pink tail pointing toward an open field just one lane away. Through studying their bodies, I had wanted to understand my own—the absence of memory, the etchings of trauma, the shape of an unseen illness. In my vulnerability, I wanted to ask someone to sit beside me, to look. I wanted to be still and splayed and open that way, to give myself over to rest. But when I most wanted to escape from my body, when I thought it had failed me beyond redemption, the farmland roads showed me that there was salt and strength left in me. On that last run down the routes I had once punished myself with, I trailed the ghost of a girl—past the cracked well, the sunken shed, the roosters still in their yard—past all the reminders of what I loved, what had held me.

I wanted to believe that running my old route one last time would be like a coda to a narrative of illness I hadn't wanted to start in the first place. One last resounding note of pain and pleasure mixed together. By returning to the site of some of my deepest grief, I could put to rest the voices of teammates whose echoes still taunted me, the terror of becoming episodic, my reluctance to accept care, and the ways I weaponized food and exercise as attempts at control. But real life is not that neat.

*   *   *

At first, Portland, Oregon, was a dream. I was starting my MFA, and my mom helped me move in. We took long, luxurious walks down a riverfront path where cormorants slipped their slick bodies beneath the surface of the water. We walked miles to find vegan cake and savored each bite of the rich coconut frosting. The city was full of potential: I could choose whom I told about what had happened to me in college or keep my history a secret, something that I thought I had left far behind me.

When my mom left, the dream of the imagined life I built dissipated. Against a backdrop that held so much potential, I was sucked down a rabbit hole of *what if.* What if, while I was miles away from my home, I collapsed on a run and disintegrated into a mess of stuttered words with no memory? What if someone found me in that state? I imagined the pressure of their hands pushing me down, lips working roughly, the metal of a zipper. Who could I call if I was in danger? My parents were moving overseas, my brother was a flight away, and Eliza and Andrea had stayed in North Carolina. The safety nets from my past—a phone number posted to the back of my iPod, a hand-drawn map left on the kitchen counter, a Post-it Note with a time I would be home—seemed worthless. They would do no good here. I attended my classes and started teaching as a graduate assistant, but instead of leaving my apartment for small outings, testing the waters of illness, I became more and more reclusive. A current of fear thrummed through my body at all hours of the day and night. I felt electric.

As I had in the months leading up to the hospital, I turned back to Freelee and Durianrider's channels. Their release from Woodstock and the associated community seemed to encourage Freelee and Durianrider to ramp up their advertising of the Raw Till 4 diet—and label new foods, like corn pasta, steamed potatoes, and lettuce, as "healthy." At the end of their video about the Woodstock incident, they revealed that they wanted to spread the word about how a high-carb vegan diet, no matter whether it was cooked or not, could have you living your happiest, healthiest life in no time. They founded the Raw Till 4 retreat, free for anyone to attend, in Chiang Mai, Thailand. "We want to make the garden bigger for everyone," Durianrider said, "not just make the garden bigger for ourselves."

Dozens of people traveled to Chiang Mai for the inaugural Raw Till 4 Thai Fruit Festival with Freelee and Durianrider in 2014. Like Benedict Lust's advertisement-in-song for the Yungborn Nature Cure in the late 1800s, attendees of the festival came up with their own smooth, sultry lyrics that they hoped would summarize their experience. The "Raw Till 4 Thai Fruit Festival (Official Music Video)" begins with an address "to all the people around the world living on fruits and healing yourselves," given by a man wearing a black fedora and a maroon, lightly patterned short-sleeved button-down. He grooves as he sings, punching his hands out in front of him to the beat, shaking his hips, pursing his lips.

So I heard that there's this thing called Raw Till 4,
eat fruits all day and maybe some more.
Then you finish off with a cooked food meal
but no other fats—that's the deal.

Chorus: It's the Raw Till 4 Thai Fruit Festival
I'm here right now and the best of all
There's so many fruit bats here too
Lovin' life, living on fruit. (Repeat)

. . . Everyone's welcome, we've got no beef
(but really, we actually don't have any beef).

Throughout the video, there's a montage of clips from the fruit festival:
shaky footage of bananas stacked at a market, vegetables heaped onto
a bed of rice, a sweaty man wrapping his mouth around the soft flesh
of a mango, a vat of what looks to be cooked quinoa, a crowd of mostly
white people wearing crop tops or no tops or "VEGAN" tops, moving
their bodies, waving bananas above their heads, lifting their own video
cameras and cell phones in the air in search of content. There are girls
dancing with mangoes, a blond person with dreadlocks, men dousing
one another with water from disposable bottles, everyone bathing
themselves in mud, people shaking their heads stiffly to the beat.
Midway through the video, the singer's voice lowers in register and
slows to a seductive drawl. "*Time to get down*," he croons. "*Move that
body, eat some durian, mangoes, mmmmm*." Two women lick each side
of a censored mango. The video ends with an invitation: "We're gonna
be here every year. We're gonna be somewhere every year, munching
on all of this glorious rainbow fruit, moving our bodies. Come along,
yeah? Everyone's welcome—and it's free."

* * *

I've never attended a Raw Till 4 Festival, visited Freelee or Durianrider in person, or even gone a whole day eating just fruit. But what I did join Freelee and Durianrider for, especially from my home in Oregon, was relief from the life I was living. My days and nights were spent preparing for teaching, which was new enough to me that I would spend hours writing out sentences like "Hi, my name is Jacqueline," so I wouldn't somehow forget. I had quit running entirely and left the house to walk to class and back and to walk to the grocery store and home. Food became something that kept me company, soothed me, filled a hunger I didn't yet know the origins of. At night, too anxious to sleep and humming with a kind of deep, abstract fear I hadn't learned to put words to, I smothered my feelings with food: entire jars of white chocolate peanut butter, enough pasta to fill a large mixing bowl, doused in olive oil and topped with an egg and spinach. I ate LÄRABARs by the dozen. I poured bowl after bowl of cereal until it felt right that I finish the box. I blended up handfuls of frozen bananas with a splash of almond milk in order to make "nice cream." Freelee and Durianrider's videos kept me company while I ate; I could watch them or any other similar influencer stuff in the calories. They used to fill their own mixing bowls with things like logs of Weetabix cereal, smashed baked sweet potatoes, diced mango, frozen blueberries, and almond milk. They would have potlucks where they brought plate after plate of carbohydrates back to their table, almost as if in competition to see who could eat the most before succumbing to bloat and fullness. They permitted consumption—in fact, encouraged it—and so again, they became a relief to me in my lowest moments, even if I wasn't following their rules.

Freelee and Durianrider, at that time, had pivoted from raw fruit to Raw Till 4-heavy messaging. In one video, Freelee adds twenty dates to a blender (for dateorade) before pouring "about half a cup" of coconut sugar in as well as English Toffee Sweet Drops® (which, ironically, on their website are advertised as being "keto-kind" for their lack of carbs). Later that same day, Freelee moves around an open field waving lettuce as if she is a ribbon dancer before tucking in to a pot of steamed potatoes at the end of the night, which she wraps in lettuce and tops with parsley and spring onions. Though Freelee clarified to her "glucose junkies" in a video that their "hair, skin, eyes" all look best on fruit, she confessed that "it feels nice to have a veggie soup or a cooked meal at night." She started eating heaping bowls of corn pasta, and Durianrider went to what appears to be a mall food court for plates and plates of brown rice and vegetables. They went out to eat low-fat curry, and poured around 100 grams (about one cup) of sugar directly into their banana and date smoothies. In the videos, they insist that what they are eating is low-fat, mostly oil-free, and limited in sodium. I asked Freelee and Durianrider to comment on whether or not they verified the food court ingredients or if they held a looser approach to their macronutrient ratios at the time, but they did not respond. Even low-fat coconut milk includes grams of fat and saturated fat—so how much was okay? If Durianrider was eating multiple servings of these foods as he indicated in his videos, didn't it add up? Footage shows heaping piles of broccoli, carrots, and sweet potatoes all mixed together—what had happened to their claims about mono-meals being easier on digestion? I don't mean to question the actual health of their diet, I only want to echo the concerns that were raised for me both back then and now as I rewatch the videos. Their platform had been built so much on the premise of purity that watching them eat in a food court with no behind-the-scenes footage of the meal preparation seemed too stark of a juxtaposition not to notice.

Though the rules of their diet had shifted, one thing hadn't: Freelee and Durianrider both emphasized that people who really followed Raw Till 4 correctly would lose weight. It was, they said (often while pinching their cheekbones or hips) impossible to be fat on a high-carb diet.

They emphasized smashing in plates upon plates of rice, enough sugar-supplemented dateorade to fill a blender, as many blueberries as there are calories in a big mac. They held up members of the community who had lost weight as examples of what their diet could do. One of these was someone who went by the username Fat2FitonFRUIT. In the beginning of the video, she is wearing a brown string bikini, standing in a nondescript room, with her hands on her stomach, yelling, "Oh my god, where did my belly button go? What you're seeing here is about a hundred thousand calories of Hungry Jack's veggie burgers, onion rings, chocolate, chippies, yeah, you get the picture."

The video cuts to her, noticeably slimmer, standing next to Freelee. The woman's identity is revealed; she is none other than Nadia, the woman who first sat next to Freelee at the raw picnic seven years before, with her pile of mangoes, and answered every single one of Freelee's questions about the raw lifestyle. "I was your teacher then," Nadia says in the video. She's wearing a colorful, striped tank top and purple leggings. "And now you've become my teacher."

Like a parody of an infomercial for a weight-loss subscription food system, Freelee and Nadia introduce proof. "Check out these 'before' photos," Freelee says.

"Be prepared to be scarred, people," Nadia chimes in.

To the tune of Florrie's "Left Too Late," the heavy-handed lyrics, "Buy a one-way ticket/ get me out of here," blaring in the background, photographs of Nadia flash onto the screen. In them, she's seated on the ground in various different bikinis, sometimes holding up a newspaper like a hostage so that the date is clear. In the "before" photos, her stomach has rolls, and in the "after," she points her toe and puts a hand on a hip, revealing a tight abdomen. To be clear, I'm not celebrating one body over another. Instead, in my opinion, Freelee's diet hinged on fatphobia, and utilized the same predatory tactics that every other diet scam does. No matter how different Freelee tried to seem, no matter how much she preached how important it was to leave society's standards behind, she was perpetuating them, and manipulating their messages until they suited what she was selling. In the beginning, I didn't blame her. But now in her fourth year as a public figure, growing a platform that supposedly was intended to proliferate the message of veganism, her responsibility seems much greater.

Plus, some people believed there was another problem with what Freelee was selling. For some people, it didn't actually work.

* * *

A question that followers had started asking on forums and through social media was: "How long did it take Freelee to lose weight?" In videos and on social media, she frequently posted "before and after" shots, but there was no clear timeline. When someone on Snapchat asked: "How long did it take you to get your vegan physique?" Freelee answered in a circuitous fashion: "It took me time to get me where I am today." She has a huge glass bowl filled with salad in front of her. "I've been vegan for almost a decade. But I saw significant improvements in my physique, you know, from the start. I gained weight—I gained over twenty pounds to start with, on this lifestyle. Things just improved in my skin a lot, in my hair, in all kinds of physical ways in my body, but yes, I did gain weight initially, and it took a couple of years for my thyroid to heal. It took time for my weight to come down."

The questions about Freelee's weight loss weren't coming from nowhere, nor were they passing curiosities. Through comments on YouTube and response videos of their own, people reported experiencing exactly the opposite of what they were supposed to. Rather than waking up lean and full of energy, the diet left them sluggish and bloated. One such person was Anna, who found the diet when she was in her first year of college. Anna had been raised on traditional Eastern European food—a lot of fermented foods, and she naturally leaned away from meat—but when she got to college, she went out to eat a lot and discovered she liked typical North American food. She gained a bit of weight and had just gotten a YouTube account, so she started browsing for alternative diets. "I knew I didn't want to do the conventional dieting where you cut calories and you exercise a ton," she told me in a Zoom interview. She found the video of Fat2FitonFRUIT's weight loss on a high-carb, low-fat, vegan diet, and was immediately interested. "This is going to seem cliché but seeing Freelee's tiny midriff in a crop top was like, whoa, that's how I want to look. I'll do whatever it takes. I was nineteen years old and I was sold."

The diet was her 2014 New Year's resolution, and she asked her family for fruit. Her dad bought her a giant box of dates, and on the first day, she made dateorade. "I remember choking on it, being like, this is so gross and overpowering," she told me in an interview. "But I forced myself to drink it because I told myself, 'This is good for me, this is what I have to do to get what I want.'" Anna's mom said that maybe she should try eating apples or grapes if she really wanted to lose weight, but Anna insisted that her mom just didn't understand the science of the diet; she was so taken with Freelee's messaging at that point that she rejected anything she didn't want to hear. She felt a strange sense of pride in being a part of the fruit community. When she went to work with her giant smoothies, she got attention. "I felt like I was doing something really, really good for myself and for the planet," Anna told me. "The more people that paid attention to it, maybe I could impart some kind of wisdom onto them."

Though Anna felt like she knew all the answers back then and trusted in Freelee, her body kept giving her signs that something wasn't right. After drinking her massive dateorades in the morning, she was exhausted. She felt lethargic and tired. As the weeks passed, she hadn't lost a pound. Instead, she recorded herself trying on clothes in September 2014: "I have nothing to wear because none of my clothes fit me," she says in the footage. Her pale skin is contrasted by the tangerine orange of the wall behind her. She is dressed in a black bra and a black skirt that cinches her upper waist so tight that small amounts of skin hang over. "I figured a good old-fashioned skirt will do. But guess what? It doesn't fit me. I bought this right around the time I started Raw Till 4 and it fit me perfectly," she tells the person behind the camera. At that point, she had been a high-carb vegan for nine months. She holds her hands up at her sides in defeat and, as a foil to Freelee flaunting the flatness of her stomach, Anna asks the person behind the camera to film the bloated slope of her frame. In another clip from her time on the diet, she leans back in an office chair to relieve the pressure from her distended stomach and says that she ate seventeen bananas and five or six cups of frozen raspberries that day. After consuming such massive quantities of fruit, she would "sit there, clutching [her] stomach like an idiot, feeling very, very sick." Anna was eating what Freelee recommended; she was smashing in the calories.

It might seem like, at this point, nine months into a diet that had the opposite effects of what was promised, Anna might stop—especially since finding fresh fruit in Canada year-round wasn't the easiest (Anna once purchased three boxes of mangoes, only to have them all rot just a few days later). But instead, Freelee's use of buzzwords like "healing metabolic damage" and telling people that things got worse before they got better kept Anna engaged. In her e-book, *The Raw Till 4 Diet*, Freelee says that "short-term weight gain is quite common, depending on your background." Freelee claims that weight gain on the diet can be a product of "bone density," as when "your body heals the density and weight of your bones will increase" or water weight, as your "cells," on the diet, go "from raisins back to grapes!" In my opinion, the way she writes about weight loss is contradictory. On one page she writes, "Ladies throw out your scale and focus on health instead of trying to micromanage your weight. Stop being so darn superficial and focus on health." But in a passage just two pages later, she says, "If you're overweight or obese (or on the other side, if you're anorexic or bulimic), it doesn't make you a bad person; it doesn't make you unworthy. It just means you haven't been living up to your true potential . . . yet." Between the two statements? A mirror selfie of Freelee wearing low-rise jean shorts and a lacy orange bustier, her shoulders narrow and wavy blond hair framing her cleavage.

Anna held on to the promise of the body she had always dreamed of and kept eating fruit. She heeded Freelee's teachings and told herself she was getting rid of toxicity in her body. "I was laying the groundwork before it got better," she remembers thinking. "But it never did. Never lost a single pound, and I did not feel good."

Eating is such an individual journey, influenced by belief systems, moral decisions, access, an array of health conditions, cultural history, personal preference, and so much more, that to reduce a diet to "good" or "bad" would be perpetuating the same harms caused by certain extreme fad diets themselves. I wanted to understand more about the nutritional principles at play and how they might intersect with a desire to get well, heal, or achieve the "perfect" body that so many of Freelee and Durianrider's followers were after, so I asked James and Dahlia Marin, the two plant-based dietitians, about what tools they might equip patients with when sifting through the seemingly endless amount of nutritional information on the internet. The following comments refer to health trends that they have seen on social media and from their years of work in the field and are not intended to refer to any specific person or movement.

One tool of note is perspective. As trained nutritionists who have been practicing for a decade, James and Dahlia have seen thousands of patients, read countless studies related to nutrition, and continue to invest themselves by keeping up with advancements in their field. In this way, they have an extraordinarily broad, research-based information set that allows them to notice trends and remain aware that each person is highly individual and might not respond to a certain diet the same way as someone else. James cautioned that taking the advice of someone who does not do this might be cause for concern. When a person begins proselytizing an approach to eating that works for them, you have to step back and ask: Is this based in research or their personal experience? If a diet works for one person, "You are your own case study," James shared. "That's great, but I wouldn't base anything on that."

Also important is thinking about the nutritional reality of eating a diet solely based on fruit. James mentioned that fruit today is far different from what our ancestors might have eaten hundreds of years ago. "A banana in the Paleolithic era was different," James told me. "They were stubby and small, more starchy, and they had seeds. Even if you ate ten of those, you're in no way getting the amount of sugar and flesh you're eating in a banana we see in 2023 or in this modern age." Present-day fruits are nutritious, James and Dahlia both emphasized, citing that they are great sources of carbohydrates, hydration, and a few amino acids. But to exclusively eat fruit and nothing else? Dahlia explained that there are dangers inherent, like missing out on a lot of the amino acids that our body cannot synthesize on its own. "When people think about amino acids and protein, they think muscle. It's not just about deteriorating muscle and going into that muscle breakdown. These amino acids are very important co-factors for making things like neurotransmitters," Dahlia explained. In the short term, a lack of amino acids might just cause abdominal discomfort after eating a meal high in fructose. Long-term, because of a pathway called the GLUT5 fructose transporter that requires an amino acid called tryptophan, the absorption of which is affected by consuming high amounts of fructose, the body might not be able to utilize its own stores of tryptophan as well as it should. "Tryptophan is a precursor to making serotonin, one of our neurotransmitters that helps us feel calm," Dahlia shared. "Not only does it help with our mental health and our emotional state, tryptophan and serotonin are also really important for gut motility, and serotonin is important for making melatonin, which helps us sleep.

So sure, someone might feel great for the first month [on a fruitarian diet] because they have stores of these essential amino acids, these essential nutrients that they were eating before. I hear this time and time again from my patients: 'I felt really great at first. And then I was really bloated. And then I started feeling really depressed. And then I started feeling really lethargic. And then I noticed I was having breakdown in my muscles. And then, after a couple months, my sleep became poor.'"

Lastly, James and Dahlia encourage practitioners to think about context. "There are those out on social media who drink glasses of sugar water and cane sugar and throw sugar in your smoothies and eat a bunch of fruits. It's an insane amount of sugar and carbohydrates. Are you going to use all that energy? If not, your body is not going to like it. Context matters," James emphasized. "Are you training for an ultramarathon? Are you swimming and biking and running and all these things every day? Then yeah, your body will probably use all that sugar. There's science behind that."

While all of this sounds like common sense, putting it into practice is more difficult, especially in a day and age when information comes at us from so many directions and people create platforms online that begin to look more legitimate than they might be in reality. "There's a difference between a person and a brand," Dahlia told me. "Often people will start a brand based on something and then they feel like their personality has to turn into that brand, whether it's the best for them or not." Because of the confluence of individual person and brand, melded together through curated content on social media, extrapolating nuance and acknowledging personal evolution can be difficult. If you have become your brand, how do you suddenly confess that you have changed to an audience that follows you for a very specific reason? Additionally, Dahlia notes that voices like hers and James's—they are plant-based themselves but encourage their patients to make the choices that are right for their present situations, health issues, and lifestyles—aren't as catchy as the more polarizing, extreme opinions that go viral.

"People like us who say, 'Do what you need to do for your own good and for yourself,' that's not as exciting," Dahlia told me. "People aren't going to be like, 'Ooh, I'm riled up about Dahlia.' Unfortunately, with our times, people are attracted to extremism. They are attracted to somebody saying, 'Just do this and it will fix all of your life's problems.'"

When choosing to follow someone online, Dahlia encourages people to ask: "Does this person have high emotional intelligence? And does this person live a life that I would want to live myself?" If the answers to these questions are no, it might not be the best fit. Dahlia mentioned a variety of lifestyle factors that might influence dietary choices: people who cook for a family, the deeply personal ways that trauma can affect our relationship to food, living in a city, or working long hours. It's also important to note whether the person is an expert in your particular situation; for example, a cardiologist advertising a certain diet might not be the best person to take advice from if your issue is IBS. "Ask yourself these questions before you expect yourself to carry out the things that that person is carrying out. It might not work for you, and it might not even be working for them, but you just don't know it."

*   *   *

By the time the 2015 Thai Fruit Festival rolled around, the community hadn't started crumbling publicly just yet. Instead, on day one of the festival, a video shows Freelee and Durianrider walking their bikes alongside a pond in Chiang Mai. A large tree is dappled in the sunlight of late afternoon. When the couple gets close to the crowd, Durianrider yells, "Let's get this party started!" and the people cheer in response. There's a moment early in this footage that seems metaphorical for what the group was becoming. The YouTube user who uploaded this video, Javier S., films Freelee and Durianrider from their elevated position standing next to their bikes, both have their phones out, filming the crowd back. They pan from one side to the other, as does the person filming for YouTube. In both real life at the festival and via parasocial relationships online, the group was becoming insular. Freelee and Durianrider dispensed rules, followers bounced information off one another, and all of them refuted information from the outside world. All of them filmed and posted about one another, refracting each other's images and ideas. Anna describes having "an echo chamber in that community" that allowed her to reassure herself the plan "would work eventually." The former follower who wishes to remain anonymous reflects, "As soon as I was indoctrinated with a certain mindset and paradigm, I just sought confirmatory information. I would watch vegan doctors and plant-based doctors and all the vegan documentaries, and I would watch these YouTubers who were already living this lifestyle and anyone who had anything different to say; it's really easy to find information that they're wrong."

Freelee and Durianrider cultivated an "us versus them" mentality by publicly shaming people, both in videos and in real life, who they felt had betrayed them. In the video of their welcome Q&A event by the pond, Durianrider calls out snakes in the grass. "There's some people here going, 'Durianrider and Freelee are for the ego and for the money.' And they're here in the crowd today. I don't know if you know this, but they are here today. And they hate us on Facebook, they hate us on the internet, saying, 'Your guys' message doesn't work, you guys are about the ego. You guys are about the money.'"

"Why would they turn up?" Freelee asks.

"Why the fuck would you turn up, these people?" Durianrider echoes. "There's a couple in the crowd I see. Why would you turn up to our free event and say we're about the money? You get a bunch of bananas, a bunch of perfect, organic bananas, you're always going to get a moldy one or two. That's just Murphy's Law. So a message to those moldy bananas is: We don't want ya. Some of you know who we're talking about. Why come?"

As had been the case the year before, the fruit festival was an event mostly characterized by daily group rides up Doi Suthep mountain, trips to the fruit market, endless plates of white rice and veggie-heavy curries, and a choreographed flash dance in the park performed by people wearing tank tops featuring watermelon slices or phrases like #cutcarbscutlife. But the event in 2015 was tainted by some drama. As Freelee explains in a video titled "Thai Fruit Fest Drama My thoughts and Review," "There was [sic] a few people who got involved in what I call a storm in a teacup and made it into a storm when it didn't have to be that. You know, Chinese whispers begin and people say things about others behind their back and they create something that wasn't there before, which is really disappointing. I was disappointed in some people who were involved in that."

Though Freelee is vague in her video, not naming anyone involved or even the drama itself, rumors circulated on gossip sites and through YouTube videos like a nightmarish game of telephone. The drama centered around one central issue: A man rented out a house in Thailand and let some fellow festival attendees, all of them women, stay with him. What happened next is hearsay, and the women involved have not responded to my requests for an interview, nor could I locate any videos from them online in which they spoke about the incident. The truth about the situation belongs to the women involved, who have chosen not to comment publicly, but the public perception of the event, as I've gathered from videos from various people who attended the festival that summer, is that there was an alleged incident of sexual harassment. I will not be commenting or weighing in on the veracity of these claims, as I have not independently verified them in any way. However, Durianrider's response to the incident serves as a moment of foreshadowing for what was to come. About the man who was accused of sexual harassment, Durianrider says, "[Man] touched [woman A's] hand. He grabbed it, at a restaurant. [Woman A] was saying, 'I haven't had a date in a while, my husband left me, I haven't had a date in a while,' and [Man] said, 'I'll be your date.' And he grabbed her hand. [Woman A] pulled her hand back and said, 'No.' It's fine if you have a go, [Man]. [Man], he's an alpha male, he likes pussy, and he's a businessman, like a lot of guys out there, so of course he's gonna have a go. That's the 'sexual harrassment' that occurred."

Durianrider continues by saying that he wanted to get Woman A on his channel to do an interview about the incident, but, "She didn't even reply back. Too busy reapplying makeup in the mirror. And that's fine. Doesn't make her a bad person. I don't hate [Woman A], I just see her as a young, immature, inexperienced, spoiled brat." Diminishing the alleged sexual harassment by writing off potentially predatory behaviors as "alpha male" characteristics and insulting a potential victim are alarming, but also speak to the kind of misogynistic content that Durianrider was posting regularly. He made videos like "HOT babe with flat stomach gets negged by Durianrider," where he films Freelee and tells her, "Looks like you've got a bit of a gut going on there." He posted a video where he filmed Freelee coming in and out of a changing room with an array of tiny shorts on, the camera trained on her shoulders down. For much of the three-minute footage, she is a faceless model, twirling, shaking her bum, checking the fit on each pair she tries on. At one point, while she's closing the door to the room, she looks at the camera and says something like, "Ah, you better not put this video on the internet," and Durianrider responds, "No, not at all," before chuckling to himself. Toward the end of the footage, Durianrider holds his camera up over the door to peer in on Freelee in the private changing room. She flips him off, smiling.

*   *   *

In the video Freelee made about the Thai Fruit Festival allegations, she makes a plea to her community to give up the infighting and focus on what's really important. "We look at the big picture and we see that we've got people dying around us, we've got animals dying, we've got the planet dying, and we give attention to drama," she says. "We really need to make that connection in our head and give our energy to things that really, really need our energy." What's ironic about her asking for peace is that she herself became an instigator. She didn't make videos only about animal rights, compassionate living, or finding creative solutions for veganism in far-flung places. Instead, as revealed in an interview for a *Jezebel* article published in 2016 by Ellie Shechet, Durianrider recalls coaxing Freelee into creating more controversial content. "Not many people can handle the drama," Durianrider told Shechet. "I remember Freelee at the start couldn't handle it and I said look, this is really good for views." (Freelee didn't dispute this claim.) The clickbait ranged from Freelee calling out trending celebrities—"Kim Kardashian makes me sad," "Rihanna is blood-thirsty and EVIL? (Warning Graphic)," "Khloe Kardashian's diet and lifestyle habits," "Cara Delevingne Weight Loss Secrets REVEALED," and "Taylor Swift Secret to staying skinny REVEALED"—to Freelee blaming a person's death from cancer on chemotherapy, to saying, "When your obese brothers and sisters get stuck on the stairwell on 9/11 preventing fit people from getting through and surviving, you make it part of my business."

Some followers defended Freelee's aggressive internet persona by saying that the end goal (saving the animals) was worth the means. But others began to point out the hypocrisy in Freelee living a "compassionate" life while trolling and demeaning other women in her videos. In the comments on her video "Why did Selena Gomez gain weight? Call me girlfriend!" user Amanda S. writes, "I don't think these videos are helping attract more people into the lifestyle, just creating controversy," while others, like welshcorgiluv, point out, "You can't just fucking say she's 'addicted to stimulants' over a few pictures of her holding a fucking coffee cup." Others noted that Gomez had been diagnosed

CHAPTER 16

A Different Kind of Garden

BACK AT THE FIRST FARM GATHERING IN CAIRNS, THINGS seemed so simple, so good. The people ate from the land: the green lily pad leaves of tatsoi, cherry tomatoes, and sweet leaf straight from the stalk. They cleaved open sugarcane just to taste something sweet. They were vegan for the animals. They were vegan to heal themselves from the harms they had put their bodies through in the past. They spoke gently to one another. They had found a path that felt good to them, and they wanted others to feel good, too. That was all.

Maybe I am simplifying the origins of Freelee and Durianrider's—Leanne and Harley's—journey. But when I look back on the videos that they posted in 2009, I see them sitting across a table from each other, feasting on durian. I see Durianrider at the market, separating the flesh of a mammal from the flesh of fruit. I see grainy footage of produce laid out on a rug, Freelee softly complimenting the taste and look of each organized pile. I see two people who had come from histories of substance abuse, unhealthy relationships, disdain for themselves, frustration with the ways medical systems had failed them. I see what must have seemed like a series of the kinds of miracles each of us might dream of—first, the fruit that healed them, then a connection between them, a love for each other that was made stronger through their commitment to the animals and the earth. I wonder—almost hope—that there was a point in their relationship where they did live in a kind of Eden of their own, one that held them and allowed them a taste of paradise, even if just for a moment.

In life, and in this story, there is no one forbidden fruit to refrain from, no one serpent whispering something dangerous.

After being kicked out of Woodstock, Freelee and Durianrider tried to brand their festival as being inclusive. They would welcome every high-carb vegan under the sun. They wouldn't kick you out for eating a boiled potato! They were reasonable! Their event was free! And if you biked to the top of the mountain each morning, you were guaranteed to get time with the gurus themselves, a generosity of wisdom and time that not everyone was willing to give. Their goal was to build their event to be the biggest it could be, so their "carbed-up soldiers" could show the masses that veganism—specifically high-carb veganism—was the way. But in the buildup to the 2016 Raw Till 4 Festival, videos posted to Durianrider's YouTube account started to show cracks in the facade. In one video, breaking open the carefully curated image that Freelee posted to the internet, Durianrider secretly films her. She's sitting in bed, leaning against the backboard, a hand resting lightly on her stomach. She's eating boiled potatoes straight from a stainless steel pot, smacking her mouth enough that pieces fall onto the bed beside her. When she realizes she's being filmed, there's a moment where I feel tender toward her. She asks, "What are you doing?" before trying to loosen her hair from behind her ears so that it better frames her face. She throws her hands up in front of her and says, "Leave me alone. No cameras." Durianrider concludes by lifting his finger so it's just in frame. He points to her stomach. "Touch the potbelly," he says. He pairs the footage of Freelee eating next to a frame of a pig grunting in front of a camera, noisily scarfing down a potato chip placed in front of its snout.

In another, Durianrider revealed just how far he had fallen from his certifiably raw life. In a "What I Eat in a Day"-style video posted March 28, 2016, Durianrider chronicles consuming a few sips of Freelee's two-liter orange juice (prompting a "fuck you very much" from an off-camera Freelee); two Clif bars, one of which contains caffeine ("Be wary of that, they'll give you a buzz," Durianrider says); a bowl of glassy-looking sweet potato noodles, featuring a bit of Arrabbiata sauce; four cheese-free pizzas from Domino's; and, for dessert, some vegan vanilla ice cream from the carton and a two-liter bottle of orange Sunkist ("No artificial colors or flavors, just sugar and water," Durianrider clarifies). It strikes me, while watching, that it seems like Durianrider doesn't just give himself permission to enjoy these foods freely. Instead, through comments like "sugar and water," he orients these meals and judges their value around the rules he had formerly created for himself. I can imagine that, after creating a livelihood based around a specific diet, it would be hard to let it go, and to worry then about how followers would receive it. In that way, I empathize deeply when I watch this video. But in other ways, I think there's a level of responsibility someone has when they have a platform based around food, particularly when they have given people around them rules based on beliefs that, to my knowledge, are not supported by specific degrees or supervised training in nutrition.

*   *   *

At the start, I thought of Freelee and Durianrider as Adam and Eve: two fallible people tempted by the same lure of perfection, youth, and health that is sold to all of us in some way or another.

As I wade further into the weeds, the metaphor deteriorates. For as Freelee and Durianrider welcomed more followers into their garden, as they continued to promise a kind of body that did not always come to fruition, they continued ratcheting up their sense of control through a series of convoluted rants and rules. Followers who did not comply were expelled from the garden forever. Henya Von Perez says she was one of them; she was banned from the Facebook group, and many committed Raw Till 4 members shunned her as a result, demeaning her in videos, lamenting about her diet choices, or portraying her as a money-hungry influencer who had infiltrated their group for some easy cash because she had sold T-shirts that said "#CUTCARBSCUTLIFE" at the Raw Till 4 Festival. (Flying to Thailand to eat large quantities of carbs and sell a few T-shirts doesn't seem like the most glamorous or lucrative of money heists, but to each their own.)

The bannings didn't stop with just Henya. Instead, as Durianrider describes in two separate videos, one of them archived by a YouTuber named Jackson (username Plantriotic), the history of the fruit festivals went like this: "That first year we had was the Thai Fruit Festival. We had a lot of shit cunts come to that, a lot of space cadets," he says. Durianrider holds his hand up, twinkles his fingers, and makes his voice breathier and higher. "Ahhh, breatharian, fruitarian, just space cadets. Then we had the 2015 Raw Till 4 Thai Fruit Festival and we got less shit cunts, more cyclists." This year, he wanted something different. "We don't want 'drainbows' with a gratitude deficiency, self-entitled rich kids, spongy fucking energy time-vampires who go, 'Biking up here is stupid. I'm coming to Chiang Mai because I want to be like a fucking shit cunt.' That's not who we want . . . These people mistake kindness for weakness, so we're gonna raise the bar. It's like a skinny-tea detox shit cunt purge just using water and carbs and truth."

Just two months before the 2016 Raw Till 4 Festival was to begin, Durianrider and Freelee changed the rules of who could participate. They purged their group of all the "drainbows" by deleting the old Facebook group, one that had 12,000 members but was "diluted" in their eyes. They made a new group. In order to join, you had to have a Strava account. When added to the Facebook group, you had to post a photo of yourself on a bike with a "V" sign in the air. Some followers who had planned to attend, like Jackson and his girlfriend, Izzy, were disappointed that they had spent such large chunks of time and money planning for a festival that they were now banned from. Both seemed like the ideal candidates for the festival: Izzy had 50,000 subscribers on YouTube, Jackson had a bike chain tattoo and a "Carb the Fuck Up" tattoo framed by a banana on his foot, and both cycled. But it wasn't enough. They weren't allowed into the new, exclusive Facebook group. Not only that, but they felt Durianrider, who they had long looked up to as a vegan role model, shamed them. To a then-nineteen-year-old, Durianrider (who was thirty-nine at the time) wrote, "@izzythatfruitbat don't come to our events mate. We have a shit khunt free policy this year. #thanks." When Durianrider described the new order of things on camera, he became so passionate that spittle gathered at the corners of his mouth. "Go and do some flake fest," he advises followers who have been ejected from the group. "Smoke heaps of bongs and rent a bike and blow your life."

The false dichotomy Durianrider sets up between followers who cycled and those who didn't came as something of a surprise. Sure, followers had cycled up Doi Suthep in the past, and many people who attended the Raw Till 4 fest had brought their bikes along, but those who didn't were free to create their own activities: dance lessons, language classes, concerts, and outings to nearby attractions. Suddenly, their lack of interest in cycling, even if they were hardcore high-carbers, meant that they should just give up the lifestyle and go smoke some weed. One hopeful Thai Fruit Fest attendee, Lex, who preferred jiu-jitsu to cycling, confronted Durianrider about his video at the Los Angeles VegFest and filmed the encounter. "What would you say to us shit cunts who do not cycle but wanted to go to the Thai Fruit Festival?" she asks. Durianrider smiles and rocks back and forth on his heels. He responds, "I did that much more as a safety thing, because last year there were a lot of crashes so I created a bit of controversy so people would start talking about it and maybe ride a bike more and be safe in Thailand." He tells Lex that she can attend, and that she's welcome to walk to the top since she doesn't bike. What I find interesting about this situation is the insight it gives into Durianrider's YouTube strategy—controversy, he seems to feel, is more effective than simply distributing information via any one of his platforms—as well as the noticeable difference between his demeanor behind his own camera—laden with profanity and insults—and the calm, rational answer he offers Lex when she asks him the question behind her own. For a few followers, Durianrider's initial video was the wake-up call they needed to separate themselves completely from Freelee and Durianrider and explore the world of veganism on their own, with more nuance. But for others, the 2016 Raw Till 4 Festival was the peak of their experience before the group came crashing down.

*   *   *

The candy-coated version of the Raw Till 4 Festival in 2016 had a remix of OMI's "Cheerleader" in the background. At the moment the trumpets blare into being, influencers started cycling up Doi Suthep, singing "Ohhh, we're halfway there" with friends. They had deep conversations while rolling out their muscles after the ride. They made a trip to the mall to gather jackfruit and boxes on boxes of cereal. ("Oh, I think that I found myself a cheerleader.") They ate plates of white rice, steamed sweet potatoes, corn, and lettuce, topped with a little drizzle of Sriracha. They went to dinner at Taste From Heaven, a vegan and vegetarian restaurant, to eat papaya salad, pumpkin curry, green soup, and a large chocolate brownie for dessert. They ate until they had to lean against the wall for support, until they had to lie back, let their stomachs see the light, and put sunglasses on as if hungover ("I'm like a little bit food coma," one of the influencers says). At home, they smashed two liters of water, and adhere "CARB THE FUCK UP!" stickers to their bikes. One of the influencers sat down with a large mixing bowl of cereals and fruit, and all the friends shared a laugh over how much they said "mmm" in any given day. They did it all again the next day and the next. On video, their days include a flurry of Disney songs they belt out at any given moment; heaps and heaps of mixed, high-carb cereal with sugar poured on top; the *best* jackfruit they'd ever had, the *best* mango, the *best* friends, the *best* time.

From where I sat, thousands of miles away, watching, it did look like the best time. It looked full of color and laughter and fresh fruit and trim bodies in bikinis. It looked like the opposite of my life. In Portland, I felt perpetually frantic, like a rat trying to escape a cage. I did not understand yet that I was the cage. The months I'd spent lying in counseling, years spent avoiding counseling, and otherwise not dealing with the loss of the cross-country team, my teammate pressing his weight down onto me, the echoes of former friends' cruelty and the way that a non-diagnosis left me in a convoluted limbo with myself—all of it meant that I feared what my body would do in any given situation, and also what others might do to me.

I had a recurring nightmare that started after I got sick and stayed with me for years; it's maybe a better way of saying how I felt than I could ever admit otherwise. In the nightmare, I am at a house with my old cross-country team. An oversized blue blow-up pool with a slide is in the middle of the yard. A male teammate I had dated freshman year is sitting on a roof with his new girlfriend, but everyone else, including me, vacillates between running around the backyard and swimming. Out of nowhere, it seems, soldiers march to the fringe of the yard and order us to all get in the pool. Guns glint in the bright summer sun. Everyone laughs at the guards except for me; I see a rope ladder attached to the roof, so I start climbing, hoping someone will save me. When I grip the gutter and hoist myself onto the roof, the new girlfriend starts laughing at me. I say, *stop, stop, do you see the guards?* And she laughs. Peals of laughter echo from the yard, the whole team staring up and laughing at me. Terrified, I jump off the roof and into the shallow pool, my legs absorbing the impact. Everyone is still laughing when a soldier shoots me in the stomach. When I look down, there is a gaping hole in my torso. *I need someone,* I scream, my throat raw. *Help! Can't you see the men?* No one responds, so I get out of the pool, my clothes heavy and drenched. I try to run down the hill, toward the trees and away, but my legs won't respond to my commands: *let's go, we need to go, we need to run.* At the end, I am still trying to run, a cacophony of laughter swallowing me whole.

After leaving the team, I had wanted to believe that their cruelty toward me did nothing. I wanted to pretend that because I couldn't actively remember most of the bad parts, it meant that they did not exist. But when I started writing about my experiences for my MFA program, they felt like sharp glass, painful to pick up and look at for long. I could not yet shape the memories; they emerged raw, without commentary, and without the grace of hindsight that falling in love and learning to run again and allowing myself to feel the pain of those college days in safe spaces and a decade of friendship with Eliza and Andrea would bring. I spent much of that year feeling like I was hurting myself by thinking about the past but needing to all the same. Portland, to me, was signing up for a marathon and being too afraid to even jog a mile; it was staying in bed on race day, while the runners made their way down the road near my apartment. Portland was all grey skies and the hum of something unnameable that felt wrong and the compulsion to eat more and more and more until my stomach was taut with a sharp pain, until finally my anxiety dulled in comparison, even if it was just for a little while.

With me in that darkness—and releasing me from that darkness— were the fruit bats halfway around the world, whose lives I coveted, whose technicolor videos of waterfalls and abundant fruit and sureness in their beliefs covered up a different reality: that they, too, carried doubt, and they, too, were haunted by illnesses that, in some cases, would soon eclipse them.

*   *   *

On the last day of the Raw Till 4 Festival, not knowing it would be their final one, Freelee and Durianrider sat on a concrete podium at the top of Doi Suthep, before a crowd of their followers, to answer questions. Watching the video feels like being suspended in time, as if Durianrider will forever be wearing his "VEGAN" shirt, Freelee her "HARDEN THE FUCK UP" ball cap.

"What do you know about heart palpitations?" someone asks. The crowd is lively. People joke with one another, chatter.

"School's in session!" Durianrider says, smiling.

"We're starting," Freelee says, and she smiles too.

"Heart palpitations can be from nervousness, caffeine, stimulant usage, maybe if someone's a bit dehydrated, also if someone is new to exercise and they're not used to their heart, like, pumping hard, they might mistake it as a palpitation," Durianrider explains. Freelee sneaks a look at her phone that's tucked just behind her thigh. "It's a pretty general thing. Are you talking about yourself or what?"

"Yeah, sometimes," the person says.

"What does the heart palpitation feel like to you?" Durianrider asks. "What are you feeling?"

"It'll beat really fast?" Freelee asks. And the person agrees. "I've always had that," she says.

"It's normal," Durianrider says. "You just want to keep breathing." He tells the person to breathe from their belly and keep their blood pressure low. Freelee asks the crowd if anyone else has had heart palpitations and people say yes.

The nearly two-hour conversation roams from Tony Robbins's book recommendations, to how many followers make for a social media expert, to sore hamstrings, to how fast Durianrider is this year. At some points, there are such long pauses between questions that you can hear the sound of a rooster and birds chirping. Durianrider talks about how oil can make your red blood cells coagulate or give you oily skin or even inhibit your glycogen levels and impede recovery. Durianrider tells people his preferred energy during a ride is 100 grams of sugar mixed into a water bottle. Freelee holds her phone up and shoots a panorama of "all those happy faces," and Durianrider holds his phone up to take a similar set of photos, a reminder that they are curating content as they are dispensing it. They dream out loud about the possibility that the whole planet might go vegan in the next thirty years, if other people are sure to make "celeb videos, fitness videos, or whatever videos" instead of "videos about other vegans." With no context, Durianrider talks about how when he has a bad day, he turns the light off, rests, and thinks "about that person, somewhere in the world today, who got hit by the machete militia, lost their legs, lost their daughter, lost their mother, lost someone close to them. They were just in the field picking corn, someone comes through and chops them up because they have a different religious perspective, and then they're laying there waiting for the Red Cross that may or may not come, forever maimed for life, just believing in whatever and picking corn."

What strikes me about their answers is the absence of depth despite the pair having so much time and space to talk. Their comments and questions about heart palpitations feel like those that a medical doctor might ask, but without the training to support the reassurance that they offer. Red blood cells don't "coagulate" due to oil (in fact, olive oil might have the opposite effect). And it is unclear which "machete militia" Durianrider is referring to. I could go down a rabbit hole of every claim made in the two hours of footage, but the further I get into consuming what Freelee and Durianrider have created, I realize that this two-hour-long set is perhaps a metaphor for much of their content. The videos themselves are a kind of fruit; I've been seeking the same feeling of fullness that Anna, Bonny, Raini, and so many others have. I've been chasing the illusion that if I watch just one or two more videos, I'll finally understand who Freelee and Durianrider *really* are. I'll finally uncover whether or not they knowingly led followers into harm or whether they truly, until the bitter end, believed in the power of fruit to save and to heal. For nearly a decade now, I've been consuming this media in different forms. I'm still hungry. Maybe that's the point. There is money to be made from my clicks, from my consumption. There are profits to be made from making people believe in an illusion of the thing they want most. How much? In Freelee and Durianrider's case, I'm not sure (I reached out to Freelee and Durianrider for comment on this question, but received no answers). The tricky part about ballparking a figure is that there are too many streams of revenue that are controlled completely by Freelee and Durianrider—starting in 2012 with Freelee's $650 per month "Fruitionist" memberships. In 2020, I spent $72.95 on Freelee's self-published e-book bundle and $35.99 on Durianrider's; I would assume, because they are self-published, that the profit margin is high. Freelee and Durianrider's frequent posting on YouTube has yielded them enough to live on for over a decade, but beyond that knowledge, the figures are murky. In 2015, Durianrider made a video saying Freelee made "as much as a doctor." In 2022, he claimed she has made "millions and millions" from her different platforms.

a girl who wanted more and got angry or jealous or whatever." (I sent Harley multiple requests for comment on this issue but did not receive a response.) Durianrider accused Freelee of secretly using Juvederm, a cosmetic filler. (Freelee, on Tumblr, later posted she did use the product, explaining that her self-esteem was low while she was with Durianrider, who she claimed spoke to and about her in a "derogatory way," insisted that she wore "skin-tight clothing" and would "harass and belitte" her until she obeyed.) In the Daily Mail, it was reported that Freelee accused Durianrider of using steroids. They both alleged that the other had been abusive in their relationship. The end of Freelee and Durianrider's relationship came with tearful videos, attacks via a variety of online platforms, and followers who took sides. The end, to me, also seemed to indicate how much the couple had considered public image during their time together. The reality we see on social media isn't ever the full truth.

The public demise of their relationship wasn't the only sign of the movement's collapse. The former follower who wishes to remain anonymous, who had wholly embraced the tenants of the lifestyle—she had a thriving YouTube channel, cycled, attended two festivals, smashed in the carbs, and had a personal friendship with Durianrider and Freelee (she described Durianrider as a "soft-spoken person with a mild temperament" in person, and Freelee as "super quiet" and "really humble")—remembers that time period as holding both good and bad. To her, it felt like the "ultimate hedonistic pursuit of momentary pleasure . . . we were just trying to follow the sunshine, go where it was nice, travel, eat yummy vegan food. But at the end of the day, I don't think I had any sense of deep meaning that was created from doing this long arduous toil of putting your head down and getting through it for some long-term reward."

After the festival, the former follower continued traveling. When she returned home, she began experiencing hormonal issues that impacted her progesterone, estrogen, and cortisol levels. During the worst of her symptoms, she felt anger, both toward herself and toward Freelee and Durianrider. People who started on the diet at the same time as she did "were all starting to notice that this movement wasn't all that it was meant to be. They had certain deficiencies, or their hair was falling out, or their skin was breaking out, or their hormones were going off. Those problems all started bubbling to the surface around the same time, around the four-year mark. It was just enough time for the effects to come to fruition if you were too strict about it or limiting too many macronutrient categories. I think a lot of its demise probably correlates with the health of the people within that movement's deterioration." She found a strange kind of solace in knowing she wasn't alone.

Though she—and others—claim they were experiencing health issues, revealing those to followers didn't come without a cost. In my view, people whose bodies did not respond to the diet the same way Freelee's had were shamed for not following eating protocols properly. I've watched hours and hours of Freelee and Durianrider's YouTube videos, and I personally have not seen one where they respond to a follower's criticism of their diet protocols by saying something that indicates acceptance for a different way of eating. Instead, I have seen videos where former followers' choices were questioned. For example, in a video Freelee created in response to Anna's "Raw Till 4 (RT4) left me Fat, Broke, & Unhappy," Freelee attacks Anna's credibility. When Anna says she accumulated footage from her two years on the diet, Freelee, in a voiceover, says, "How do I know? How do we even know? We have no proof of that actually being true. You have to take it with a grain of salt." When Anna comments that she went through "a lot of bananas and a lot of expensive fruit and a lot of frustration, as you all have seen," Freelee, in a voiceover, comments, "No one said that you have to buy organic, tropical fruits from Whole Foods.

Let's get it straight, okay? That was your choice." The back and forth continues, but the details aren't the point; instead, it is interesting to think about the dynamic that these kinds of reaction videos set up. While Anna's original video now has 495,000 views on YouTube, her platform, with 2.93k subscribers, is noticeably smaller than Freelee's. Rather than encouraging feedback or open dialogue about the diet and its effects, this kind of public scene-by-scene response video, in my view, attempts to undermine Anna's credibility and experience. As the creator of this diet, Freelee's response, in my opinion, encourages people to place the blame on themselves rather than allowing for a greater freedom of experience.

This reminds me of religion in the way that doubt can be weaponized. The parallels between the insularity of this high-carb, raw vegan movement and religious communities is that people feel guilt and fear about leaving. For those who left the high-carb, raw vegan movement, there was a good chance that they would be publicly shamed by the group's leaders. "I think I kind of created this prism for myself, where I would say things with such absolute certainty," the former follower who wishes to remain anonymous told me over the phone, "and because of that, I felt like I had to live up to my own word." Social media, which had once felt like the ultimate expression of, and vehicle for, freedom, enabling influencers to travel around the world and film their lives as their work, had become a trap. Declaring publicly that you weren't high-carb anymore—or even vegan anymore, as some chose—came with consequences. Because many vegans stick to the diet for moral and ethical reasons (saving the planet, saving the animals, the belief that they are saving their bodies from illness), their fervor for the lifestyle is strong. Someone who is in the throes of illness trying to eat animal protein for a potential relief of symptoms, for example, isn't always received warmly; there's little room for nuance. Either you're vegan or you're not.

When the former follower got sick, and finally was brave enough to post for her hundreds of thousands of Instagram followers that she was "not a picture of ultimate health or happiness right now," and had started eating five avocados a day and plenty of walnut butter in an attempt to heal her hormones, it didn't go over well with some. Durianrider, who had once felt like "a brother, of sorts" to the former follower, wrote on his Tumblr: "Look how sick she looks now compared to how radiant she looked in Radelaide. Look how she looked before she came over to this lifestyle . . . Rich girls with daddy issues . . . " He didn't stop there. He made a video directly addressing her that he posted to his public YouTube. "What are you chasing?" he asks. He's walking down a street. Behind him, trees are laced with purple flowers. Birds chirp. "You want daddy's approval? Man, that's what's gotten you most of your problems. You're chasing approval from someone who doesn't want to approve of you because he doesn't even know how to live. You are putting on this persona. Why?"

While Durianrider accused her of putting on a persona, she was doing the opposite in those months of illness; she was finally releasing herself from the grip of performing online. "It's almost like I was dreaming or acting," she told me four years after leaving the movement, thinking back to what it was like to live her life on social media. "Something about putting a phone in front of you, looking at a camera constantly, gives you a really distorted understanding of who you are and how you should try to portray yourself. It made me constantly try to be the person other people saw me as and wanted me to be because I was always seeing myself through a lens. I always saw things from a third-person perspective: How would this look to other people?"

She feels a twinge of pain, too, thinking that her social media presence might have led people down a similar path as hers. "What were we thinking? Like, we're not doctors, we're not nutritionists. Why were we giving diet advice?" Her belief in the movement, and her enthusiasm for the diet for years, left her with long-lasting health issues. Of her time in the group and subsequent illness, she says, "I'm not happy I went through it, but I'm grateful for the opportunities that I had to grow from it. If I could avoid it, I'd probably avoid it, like in a future life."

*   *   *

After the breakup between Freelee and Durianrider, the gates of the garden were opened. Everyone left the space that had, at one time, given them hope: As a result of the video Leah Hodge posted concerning Dr. Doug Graham, as well as testimonials from other members of the Woodstock Fruit Festival, "a supermajority of Doug's peers . . .voted to not invite Doug back to the WFF" in September 2014. Graham disputed this, saying that the decision to leave WFF was "a mutual thing" and that his "vision of what the event could be was more educational oriented," rather than "party oriented." When I sent him a follow-up email attaching the public documents asserting he had been removed from the community and asking him to confirm, he responded, "I was dropped as a Pioneer. I am invited to attend the event should I so desire. The decision to separate myself from WFF was mutual." Graham has recently started an 80/10/10 Coaching Certification (a Level 1 Certification is available for $997), and it is still possible to fast with him in Costa Rica for prices that range from $7,500 to $9,000, airfare not included. "I've never wanted a bigger piece of the pie," Graham told me during our interview. "I've just wanted the pie to grow. I think there could be a lot more raw foodists in the world and I'm quite convinced the world would be a better place if there were."

Durianrider lives in Australia now, where he cycles, still has a fondness for spiders, and remains a high-carb vegan. According to a 2019 post, he believes that copious amounts of cane sugar are necessary for brain function and enhanced athletic performance. He has denied all

allegations of sexual assault. He is still dating Natasha, who is two decades younger than him. He posts videos titled: "If Her Back Doesn't
Need Adjusting, She Isn't The Right Girl For You" and "How much
money should you spend on women so they respect you?" In one video
titled "The Truth About Her Body & Cycling Shoes WILL Shock You,"
Durianrider films Natasha talking about her new shoes. She's wearing
pale blue leggings and her white ribbed crop top reveals her bellybut-
ton piercing. Rather than focusing on the shoes, Durianrider offers
a split-screen of Natasha's body. In footage featured on the left-hand
side, Natasha has been muted. She turns for the camera so we can see
her bum, turns back to face the camera, gives a stiff smile, and speaks,
though we can't hear a word.

Freelee has said that we are heading toward a "dystopian future"
and encouraged her followers to leave the cities for open land where
they might live in gardens of their own creation. She left Australia
for Ecuador, where she lived off-grid in the jungle with a man from
Sweden. In 2018, she authored a feminist manifesto of sorts, My
Naked Lunchbox, in which she writes (problematically, at times)
about how she has started to reject society's expectations of women
and instead forge her own path. She started making her own clothes.
At one point, she grew out her leg and armpit hair. She has since returned to Australia, where she still eats a high-fruit diet. Videos on
her Instagram, featuring Freelee in a knitted watermelon-patterned
thong bikini set, encourage followers to take up a high-sugar lifestyle
in order to "age at a natural rate that is healthy." Ads for her $39.95
The Raw Till 4 Diet e-book and $350 "7 Days of Private Consultation
with Freelee" pop up beneath posts. She still regularly creates videos
that shame women for their eating habits. In a recent video "What
I eat in a day in recovery" that strikes me as particularly upsetting,
Freelee offers commentary on food choices made by someone in recovery for an eating disorder. "This is going to be very interesting to
see what she's actually eating and whether it's going to lead to her

healing or not," Freelee says. "It's so hard for these people because they're getting advice from all the wrong places, right?" In a voiceover, Freelee watches the "What I eat in a day" footage and makes comments like, "There's no need to put crab in, that's for sure" or "The egg is not going to be any benefit at all, it'll make her feel worse." At the end of the footage, in a whispery voice, Freelee films herself typing a comment to the video on TikTok. "Hey Olima! Please check out my video I made for you on YouTube. I've got countless testimonials of people who have healed on fruit based diet!"

CHAPTER 17

How to Heal

AFTER TWO YEARS IN PORTLAND, I LEFT FOR OKLAHOMA, where I had been accepted to a PhD program. The highway from the airport to get to my new apartment stretched for miles and miles, the land ahead flat. Frail trees edged the road, so little green against all that red dirt. The sky was a weak blue. All of it was beautiful. Moving away from Oregon felt like a way to cleanse myself of memory once more. In this new place, this small, sleepy town, with its Main Street just blocks long and residents who smiled as they passed me by, I vowed I would be different. I told myself that I would be safe. I told myself that nothing would hurt me. And nothing really did—except the usual culprit: myself.

During those years in Oklahoma, my greatest satisfaction came from performing a sense of wellness—I got As in school, earned leadership positions, and tried to make it appear—through my wardrobe, a perpetual smile, and a feigned sense of competence—that I was always doing just fine no matter the stressors, assignments, or responsibilities that came my way. In reality, by the third year of the program, I was crumbling. I cried most days and tried my best to achieve perfection—in evaluations, grades, and observations—within a grueling and complicated system.

Before I grappled with any of that in a meaningful way, I signed up for a marathon that would take place in the fall of my fourth PhD year. My training felt like sharpening a blade, harsh and unrelenting. I did not give myself rest. I did not give myself easy days on soft surfaces. I did not give myself permission to slow down. Instead, as I had so many years before, I ran on aching shins. I ran dehydrated. I ran until my heart pounded wildly in my chest and my face throbbed with heat. I ran after thirteen-hour days spent on campus. I ran from the men who veered their trucks close enough that I could feel their heat. I ran with the belief that if I only moved fast enough, I could catch the girl I should have been had I never fallen ill. She was always right in front of me, like a whisper of a dream I'd lost. She taunted me: *Keep up.*

I wore my body down until my lower leg swelled to the point that even walking was painful. Something about the physicality of the injury finally allowed me to stop, to say *enough.* The holy trinity I had bowed to for so long—thinness, a sense of false worth from my splits, the illusion of control I perpetuated through strict rules around food and running—began to unravel. Perhaps I'm drawn to the myth of Adam and Eve because I identify with those first moments they found themselves outside the gates of the garden, angry at their perceived failings and no longer able to be where they thought they most wanted to be. That's the power of myth, I think, to make us long for the memory of something that maybe never really existed. For so many years, I longed to be the girl on the team, someone who belonged, racing around a bend. But the girl everyone on the team knew was just an illusion made up of the same empty smiles and laughter that had earned me friendship during my many moves. I was allowed to remain complacent in my desire for external validation, never asked to be anything outside my weekly numbers. I heeded the stern words of a coach who told me I hadn't been enough—tough enough, fast enough—instead of listening to my body.

I wanted people to like me more than I cared about liking myself. I'm glad that I was forced to break away from that life, even if I carry grief about the way that it happened.

* * *

The process of undoing the harm I had inflicted for years was circuitous and terrifying. Giving up the strictures I had placed on myself meant that some of the truths I had based my life around had to be dissolved. If I couldn't tell what foods were healthy or unhealthy, how would I know what to eat every day? If I had to live in a body that still occasionally succumbed to lost episodic hours, my head rocking on a pillow, a stuttered string of words emerging from my lips, then how would I know I was worthy of care? Strangely enough, the very movement that had once been a source of unhealthy motivation for me at the height of my disordered eating became a means of healing as well.

See, I wasn't alone in my struggle to maintain such rigidity for years and years on end, nor was I the only one who wondered if there could be a life after existing with such black-and-white views of the world. Essie Honiball grappled with similar questions for a large portion of her adult life. After meeting T. O. Honiball, she still found herself floundering in situations that had previously been comfortable to her. Because of T.O.'s role as a prominent cartoonist, they were often invited to people's homes and more formal events as well. Tired from suffering her anxiety-induced convulsions, she visited a psychologist. The psychologist encouraged her to adopt a few behaviors that would allow her to enjoy company while still sticking mostly to her safe foods. She started permitting herself to say yes to tea or coffee and allowed herself to nibble on the corner of a biscuit before hiding it in a handbag or a potted plant. T. O. helped, too. People's admiration for him and his work meant that his requests to eat fruit at dinners or events were not ridiculed. Instead, people often went above and beyond to serve both him and Essie, going so far as to make fruit sculptures for them to enjoy for dinner. After T. O. died and Essie moved into a home for elderly people, she kept food in her kitchen just for guests: the makings of small sandwiches and cow's milk for coffee and tea. I imagine that this wasn't easy for her. The echoes of a harmful lie can ring for a lifetime if you let them, and Cornelius had talked enough about the "poisons" and "toxins" in food to keep her following his experiment even after his death. I imagine that for Essie, the biscuits and cow's milk in the fridge were daunting prospects at first, despite their relative smallness in the grand scheme of things. But Cornelius had said, "NO COMPROMISE IF YOU WISH TO SUCCEED," and so these gestures are proof that, toward the end of her life, Essie was willing to balance the precarious tensions of social obligation with the stringency of her own beliefs for a chance at a wider community.

Essie wasn't the only one to loosen up her thinking. No matter where I lived or where I moved, the high-carb vegans I had started following in college could remain with me; it was one of the perks—and dangers—of the parasocial relationships I had invested so much of my time in. While I had first taken inspiration from their near-religiosity, I began to find comfort in the ways they slowly unwound from the stringent beliefs that they held. As the anonymous former follower began to incorporate animal products into her diet, she asked herself questions: "Was I being vegan because I said I was vegan to everyone and therefore had to keep that up? Was I doing it because I had pigeon-holed myself?" It was when she stopped being vegan that she realized, on her own, that she really did love the plant-based lifestyle, not just for how it made her feel or the aesthetics, but because of the ethical component of saving the planet and the animals. Her deeper motivations for returning to a plant-based lifestyle allowed her to approach it with more nuance this time. She could incorporate nut butters, beans, and donuts. She could hang out with friends and drink kombucha or chai. Online, there was no room for subtlety, no room to question why or how she was eating, or whether or not her travels were sustaining her on a deeper level. But offline, she began to grow away from the binary thinking that had held her for so long. She once wrote, "We can feel emotions that our mind may think are at odds with what should be. We can be hurt, in debt, and struggling, while reveling in every moment of life. And we can also be in paradise, roaming white sand beaches and turquoise blue seas and feel nothing at all, like a ghost haunting an empty house."

Lauren Coleman, the person who once carted giant banana smoothies to her job at the pizza shop, went to university to earn a nutrition degree because of her desire to truly understand how to eat. There, she began to recognize that eating a diet super low in fat and protein is probably unhealthy. Slowly, she changed her thinking around food. When she witnessed weightlifting friends eating packaged protein bars without a care, she thought, why don't I try? She tried canned beans rather than soaking her own, and even went through a phase where she allowed herself ice cream and cheese, foods she hadn't eaten in a long time. Through all of it, her body surprised her. "I gained a lot of muscle because I was strength training," she told me in a 2020 interview, "and I felt a lot more confident in my body than when I was obsessive." She eventually found her way back to veganism—she says if she only ate for her own health, she would be an omnivore, but her care for the environment and animals outweighs any selfish motivations—but she is much more relaxed about her diet now. She doesn't obsess over food and doesn't "strive to be the purest, cleanest vegan anymore. It's really freeing and relaxing." To celebrate being able to reflect on a different period in her life, Coleman made a silly Instagram Reel in 2020 about her banana-eating days, where she said something like, "I went on this ridiculous diet, haha, can anyone else relate?" She didn't have many followers at the time, and it got maybe twenty likes, which was fine by her. But then, a few weeks later, it was up to 100 likes. The numbers kept snowballing until the video ended up receiving around two million views and 25,000 likes. Some commenters enjoyed the post, chiming in that they, too, remembered their own banana infatuation, but others, especially after Freelee posted it to her own Instagram story, started to pick Coleman's caption apart and ask why Coleman would tear another woman down. Freelee herself commented and sent Coleman DMs before Coleman blocked her. "I guess she won," Coleman said. "I took the post down. These types of people are creating a lot of harm, and I think they do need to be called out. If people want to promote vegan as being a lifestyle of kindness and consciousness, you need to have that approach with humans as well."

Over the years, others formerly part of 30BaD or fans of Freelee's videos have opened up about the complexities of their lives. There was Raini Pachak, the teenager from Utah, who still eats an entirely fruitarian diet except for a bowl of steamed broccoli every once in a while. While Raini's eating habits might not have shifted much, he has learned not to put extra shame on himself for what he eats and has distanced himself from Freelee and Durianrider. He believes them to be misguided and some of their methods to be harmful. He is currently working on a documentary about other fruitarians and appreciates getting to see that "everyone has their own slightly different approach to everything and it works for them."

There was Bonny Rebecca, a formerly vegan influencer who now eats animal products and talks candidly about what that means to her, despite pushback from other vegans on social media and YouTube.

There was Anna, who could not see the harm in her fruitarian diet despite her perpetual exhaustion, who went to Europe for a summer and one day realized how absurd it was that she had lined ten bananas up on a shelf in her hostel rather than eating the local food available to her on vacation. That summer, she biked, ate a plant-based vegan lifestyle, and didn't look much at YouTube because she didn't have the opportunity, and she came home feeling better than ever. It was enough to wake her up, and she made the video "RT4 [Raw Till 4] left me Fat, Broke, and Unhappy," which Freelee responded to via a video on her channel five years later. Still, Anna has empathy for both Freelee and people who fall prey to the diet. "I do sympathize for girls who are in their teen years and early twenties feeling like they need to look a certain way."

I, too, began to recognize that a cure is different from healing. One is a quick fix, something to mask symptoms, and the other is a deeper, often disruptive process that asks a person to acknowledge and work to remedy the real issue at hand.

For me, that meant acknowledging that I had a medical condition and unpacking the embarrassment I felt around that. It meant, with the encouragement of a professor, registering for disability services for the first time during my PhD after so many years of pretending like I was fine to push through, both in class and out. It meant saying out loud to a nutritionist that I feared I wasn't eating enough and asking her for help. It meant attending weekly meetings where I sat on the couch and petted her dog while she talked me through my fears and guilt and misguided attempts at controlling my life and my symptoms through food. It meant challenging myself: eating cereal every day for breakfast for a week, relearning to incorporate peanut butter into my diet, saying yes to going out. It meant naming what had happened to me in college as sexual assault. It meant going to therapy weekly, for years.

My life now is not set to the beat of electronic music or a crescendo of trumpets, and I'm glad for that. I still have episodes occasionally, though I've learned more about how to manage them over the years. I have done the work to see my symptoms not as bad or something to be guilt-ridden over, but instead as brief experiences. I have a partner who makes sure I feel safe, who reminds me that love is possible even—and especially—in moments of great vulnerability if I remain brave enough to open myself to it. I still run, sometimes slowly enough to watch the birds in spring flit through budding trees, and sometimes with a group of people that I have grown to trust. It feels strange and beautiful to be part of a different kind of team.

Healing is still ongoing. It probably always will be. The forces that once held me in their grip are the same ones that have existed for centuries, even if asses' milk and grapes proselytized through pamphlets and word of mouth have mutated to ads on Instagram that beckon me to inject my diet with superfoods or cleanse my gut with juice shots. Scammy cures have been here since the beginning of time and will continue to exist for as long as people do, but the more we can work to make our systems of healing more equitable for people, no matter race, gender, class, sexual orientation, or body size, the less people will get caught up in harmful practices that end up hurting them in the end.

*   *   *

I've mostly fallen away from the fruit diet now. I don't actively follow anyone who shares their high-carb mukbangs or preaches about the power of purity. In some ways, life without them feels like the dissipation of a fever dream. But perhaps not everything has truly dissolved. The memories of the years I spent with them, even virtually, have stayed with me, like the vacant shells of cicadas clinging to a tree. They remind me of who I might have been had circumstances been different. Essie Honiball, in particular, feels like my foil; the example of another life I might have lived. I see so much of myself in who Essie was, in the ways that she tried to keep herself safe from harm by withholding what she thought was sinful from her body, by consuming so much that was sweet. I wonder if Essie believed she had a choice or not. I wonder how much of the fruit diet became hers, and how much she was guided by the idea that if she was good enough, if she kept her body pure, that she would somehow be enough for Cornelius—or even for herself. As a single woman in South Africa who had been spurned by her first love and left by another, as a patient who had been harmed by the hands that were supposed to heal her, and as a person who could no longer find herself in the waters that had held her for much of her life, she held power over what she put in her body.

While it is easy for me to think of Essie as being trapped in black-and-white thinking, she was more complicated than that. At the conclusion of her own book, she rejects the very idea that fruit alone is a cure for anything, or that the path to healing is linear. "As long as there was any trace of hatred, intolerance, vindictiveness, depression, or negative criticism in my heart," she writes, "I could not expect the fruit to correct that too. I also had to work at these things . . . Even today, after all the years of work, I am in every respect imperfect."

Acknowledgments

AS MUCH AS BOTH WRITING AND RUNNING SEEM LIKE SOLITARY
endeavors, they're not. While writing this book, I have felt so lucky to
have innumerable people cheering me on. What follows is my attempt
to list a few of them, but know that if you have offered a kind word
or asked me about my story, you are in these pages too.

This book would not exist without the generosity of the many
people who let me into their lives and shared their experiences and
expertise through interviews. I know that it is not always easy to
reflect on the past, especially over the phone or Zoom with a person
who sent you an email out of the blue, so please know that I hold you
in deep gratitude, and that my life has expanded in so many ways
because you shared your stories. A special thank you to Anoeschka
von Meck, Essie Honiball's biographer, who provided extraordinarily
useful context for me to better understand Tannie Essie's story.
Anoeschka, your voice messages on WhatsApp so often brimmed
with as much kindness as they did information and were such bright
spots during a difficult time. Thank you also to the many librarians
I reached out to over the course of interviewing, all over the world,
who searched through their archives and collections for information,
answered questions about local geographies that otherwise would

have remained mysteries to me, and scanned pages that I thought were lost to history.

It was deeply important to me, as I wrote this narrative, to write from a place of empathy and to write in search of the truth, while acknowledging how complicated both truth and memory can be. The memoir sections I wrote from memory, but I utilized medical reports and interviews with family and former teammates to include more nuanced details, as well as raise questions about my own foggy perceptions of the past. In the narrative nonfiction sections, everything quoted comes directly from a source (an interview, legal documents, newspaper articles, archival materials, archived websites, books, public YouTube videos, public Instagram accounts, etc.) as listed in my notes and has been fact checked. Thank you to my fact checker, Hilary McClellen, for raising questions about small details that made big differences, locating second, sometimes third supporting sources for information I wanted to make sure to confirm, and providing such reassurance, warmth, and a stash of chocolate bars (!) as we worked together.

Thank you, beyond measure, to Kate Johnson who believed in this story from the beginning, has been there through rejection and with me in celebration, and who has the most fruitastic pun game I've ever witnessed. Thank you to Athena Bryan who saw what I was trying to do in this book and helped me get there, and to Kirsten Reach, who shepherded this manuscript to its final form through editorial notes that were an art form of their own. Thank you to Carl Bromley, and the rest of the Melville House team, including Sammi, Ariel, Maya, Madeleine, Janet, Sofia, Mike, and so many others, whose enthusiasm kept me going through the home stretch. I cannot thank you all enough for championing this book, for seeing the beauty in the story, and for reflecting it back to me in new and energizing ways.

Thank you to my teachers (Ms. Kisler, Mr. Chamberlain, Drew, Kevin, Cassie, Dr. Schwind, Paul, Apricot, Sarah Beth, Janine, too many more to list!). I have your voices of encouragement in my head when I sit down to write and your comments telling me to push further—you knew when I was capable of more, and often understood what I was trying to do before I knew exactly what to name it. In a similar vein, I thank my students, present and past, who have learned alongside me, keep me curious about the world, and remind me that there is room for play in every practice. To my colleagues, whose encouragement feels as bright as the bouquet of fruit balloons left in my office when I first got the deal, and who have advocated for space and resources for my writing. To my peers, thank you for sharing workshops with me, for commiserating about difficult drafts-in-progress, for your enthusiasm, and for hearts in the margins. And to all the writers who revealed to me what was possible by taking leaps on the page of their own, who read endless query letter drafts, who connected me with resources, and have shared their own experiences with me, I cannot begin to express my gratitude.

To my Maintenance Page pals, I am grape-ful to each of you for your love and support—fingers crossed we like this one! To my Wednesday Knights and West Chester Running Company friends, I hope you know how much you mean to me after reading this; through your kindness, your shoutouts, the laps we've shared, the bad dad jokes, and your belief in me, you have restored my love for the sport and an idea of team in a way I didn't think possible. Andrea, our friendship has felt like an extended version of our Asheville camping weekend. Courtney, I couldn't have made it through without our weekly calls, our endless Venmo coffee circuit, and the way you have always been there for me at a moment's notice. Eliza, you are the carrot hotline taped to the back of an iPod Mini. Tell those girls eating enchiladas in the dining hall that we made it.

And, thank you to my family. This is for Patricia, who saw me in a way not many others have, and for Jack, who gave me a mirror. Megan, your encouragement is as bountiful as a 5-gallon bucket of figs. Erik,

Notes

Prologue: Genesis

1. **Before the defamation lawsuit** . . . Sean Fewster, "SA court told fitness guru Kayla Itsines and Freelee the Banana Girl have settled their defamation stoush without trial," *The Advertiser,* March 31, 2015. www.adelaidenow.com.au.

2. **cups of coconut sugar poured into banana smoothies** . . . Freelee the Banana Girl, "What I ate today on a high carb diet." YouTube video, 5:28, July 24, 2013. www.youtube.com.

3. **sexual assault allegations** . . . Ellie Shechet, "A Year of Bananas, Vasectomies, and Rape Allegations With the Vegans of YouTube," *Jezebel,* November 2, 2016. www.jezebel.com.

4. **Acne covered the woman's face** . . . **Her gut was inflamed and her vision blurred, a symptom of systemic candida** . . . Freelee The Banana Girl, Go Fruit Yourself: How I Lost 40 LBS on a Raw Food Lifestyle & Regained My Health (Self-published), 8.

5. **The man, whose father had passed from cancer** . . . Freelee The Banana Girl, "Rawfood Vegan Retreat in Australia!" YouTube video, 9:58, December 13, 2009. www.youtube.com.

6. **sick of the lies. Sick of the fries** . . .**dollar$ in their eyes** . . . Harley Johnstone, *Carb the Fuck Up: Follow Your Heart With No Fucks Given* (Self-published, 2014), 9.

7. **the bad food they called Murder, Torture** . . . **and Harm** . . . Freelee, *Go Fruit Yourself,* 59, 84, 89.

8. **Junk** . . . Johnstone, *Carb the Fuck Up,* 9.

9. **Abundance of fruits and greens** . . . Freelee, *Go Fruit Yourself,* 17.

10. **They ate dozens of bananas per day** . . . Ellie Shechet, "A Year of Bananas, Vasectomies, and Rape Allegations With the Vegans of YouTube," *Jezebel,* November 2, 2016. www.jezebel.com.

11. **Dragonfruit** . . . Freelee The Banana Girl, "How much fruit I eat in a day on Go Fruit Yourself," YouTube video, 3:12, September 18, 2011. www.youtube.com.
12. **Peaches** . . . Freelee The Banana Girl, "How I stay Skinny AND Healthy all year round (music video)," YouTube video, 2:13, July 28, 2015. www.youtube. com.
13. **Papaya** . . . Freelee The Banana Girl, "Weight loss foods & piranhas?? What I ate today," YouTube video, 9:50, May 17, 2015. www.youtube.com.
14. **Mangoes, dragonfruit, persimmons, oranges, peaches** . . . Freelee, *Go Fruit Yourself,* 10, 44, 66, 72.
15. **Piles of durian crowned the man's bed** . . . Durianrider, "why they call me durianrider? #3," YouTube video, 0:06, June 26, 2008. www.youtube.com.
16. **Squishy** . . . Freelee The Banana Girl, "Epic Date Haul on 30 bananas a day!" YouTubevideo, 2:35, April 18, 2012. www.youtube.com.
17. **Created a website** . . . Harley Johnstone and Leanne Ratcliffe, "30 Bananas a Day." *30 Bananas a Day.* Accessed August 9, 2022. Archived at www.wayback-machine.com.
18. **Invited their followers** . . . **No one snuck down the road for a hamburger** . . . Freelee The Banana Girl, "Rawfood Vegan Retreat in Australia!" YouTube video, 9:58, December 13, 2009. www.youtube.com.
19. **Flab to fab** . . . Johnstone, *Carb the Fuck Up*, 11.

Chapter 2: Edenburg

1. **She taught classes like "Fundamentals of Rhythm"** . . . Anne K. Ross, "A Rhythmic Activities Camp in South Africa," *Journal of Health, Physical Education, Recreation*, vol. 25, no. 1 (1954): 24.
2. **Avid swimmer and diver** . . . Anoeschka von Meck (author, Essie Honiball's biographer), in discussion with the author. February 9, 2020 to June 14, 2022 via WhatsApp.
3. **Flowering jacaranda trees that bloomed purple** . . . Anton C. van Vollenhoven, "The History of Jacaranda Trees in Pretoria," *The Heritage Portal*, last modified January 6, 2022. www.theheritageportal.co.za.
4. **Essie had developed tuberculosis** . . . Essie Honiball, *I Live on Fruit* (South Africa: Essence of Health, 1981), 13.
5. **"Let me give you a hand, Granny** . . . Honiball, *I Live on Fruit*, 33.
6. **A picture of Essie from this time is haunting** . . . Klein, Dave. "Author of 'I Live on Fruit,' Essie Honiball dies at age 89," *The Frugivore Diet*. Accessed February 2, 2020. www.thefrugivorediet.com.
7. **The doctor who attended to her was brilliant** . . . Anoeschka von Meck (author, Essie Honiball's biographer), in discussion with the author. February 9, 2020 to June 14, 2022 via WhatsApp.
8. **When Essie was just a child in Edenburg, South Africa** . . . Anoeschka von Meck (author, Essie Honiball's biographer), in discussion with the author. February 9, 2020 to June 14, 2022 via WhatsApp.
9. **Cornelius, at seventy-six** . . . Honiball, *I Live on Fruit*, 12.
10. **Formulating his "hypothesis"** . . . Honiball, *I Live on Fruit*, 12.

11. **"fate probably decreed that when the experiment was ready to be conducted . . ."** Honiball, *I Live on Fruit*, 12.

12. **On the day of their first meeting** . . . Anoeschka von Meck (author, Essie Honiball's biographer), in discussion with the author. February 9, 2020 to June 14, 2022 via WhatsApp.

13. **"Wasting away like a diseased plant"** . . . Honiball, *I Live on Fruit*, 13.

14. **On the first day of the diet** . . . Honiball, *I Live on Fruit*, 13-14, 24.

15. **She dropped to a weight of sixty-nine pounds** . . . Honiball, *I Live on Fruit*, 14, 29.

16. **"obsession"** . . . Honiball, *I Live on Fruit*, 14.

17. **"totally unheard of, both socially and scientifically"** . . . Honiball, *I Live on Fruit*, 12.

18. **"patriarchal"** . . . William Shurtleff and Akiko Aoyagi. History of Vegetarianism and Veganism Worldwide (1430 BCE to 1969), 107. Lafayette, CA: Soyinfo Center, 2022.

Chapter 4: Fleshless, Bloodless, and Poison-Free

1. **"[No] resistance, of whatever kind, would have stopped [Cornelius]"** . . . Honiball, *I Live on Fruit* (South Africa: Essence of Health, 1981), 13.

2. **Valkenberg Naturopathic Hospital** . . . "Manslaughter Appeal Fails: Naturopath Guilty." *THE NEWS*. December 7, 1931, vol. XVIL, no. 2,617.

3. **Second of six sons** . . . "Melt Van Der Spuy Dreyer 1848-1900 – Ancestry®." 1848-1900 – Ancestry®. Ancestry.com. Accessed September 12, 2022.

4. **played football and tennis** . . . Cornelius Valkenberg de Villiers Dreyer, *The Bible of Nature and the Book of Wisdom* (Sydney: "Dynamic Plus," 1936), 244.

5. **In 1901, when he was around 19** . . . "Crown Case Closes in Trial of Naturopath," *The Herald* (Melbourne, Victoria, Australia), July 24, 1931. nla. gov.au.

6. **In 1916, at the age of thirty-two** . . . "Robert De Villiers DREYER," The AIF Project. www.aif.adfa.edu.au.

7. **Handwritten records from a visit to an MD in 1917 describe him as having a "moderate ability"** . . . Handwritten I.S.G.S. 5th MD report on "Cornelius Valkenburg De Villiers Dreyer Otherwise Robert de Villiers Dreyer," n.d., National Archives of Australia PP14/1, series number 4/3/226, control symbol PP14/1, National Archives of Australia, online. www.recordsearch.naa.gov.au.

8. **A newspaper article from 1918 mentions that "Cpl. [Corporal] Robert Devilliers Dreyer, South Africa" was wounded** . . . "Australians in Action: W.A. Roll of Honour," Kalgoorlie Miner (Kalgoorlie, Australia), June 25, 1918. www.trove.nla.gov.au.

9. **AIF records show he returned to Australia in 1919** . . . "Robert De Villiers DREYER," The AIF Project. www.aif.adfa.edu.au.

10. **He purchased 334 acres** . . . "Agricultural Bank Act, 1906, And Amendment Acts," *Government Gazette of Western Australia* (Perth, Australia), May 19, 1922. www.legislation.wa.gov.au.

11. **Melbourne . . .** Crown Case Closes in Trial of Naturopath," *The Herald* (Melbourne, Victoria, Australia), July 24, 1931. www.nla.gov.au.

12. **Body needed to be purified from "sin" . . .** Dreyer, *The Bible of Nature and the Book of Wisdom*, XVI.

13. **Herman Carl Arnold, who, in 1931, was fifty-five years old and a salesman . . .** "The Naturopath Hospital: Death of Cancer Patient," The Age (Melbourne, Victoria, Australia), November 10, 1931. www.nla.gov.au.

14. **If Cornelius's book,** *The Bible of Nature*, **is any indication of his methods . . .** Dreyer, *The Bible of Nature and the Book of Wisdom*, 16-17.

15. **Arnold had something wrong with his spine . . .** "The Naturopath Hospital: Death of Cancer Patient," *The Age* (Melbourne, Victoria, Australia), November 10, 1931. www.nla.gov.au.

16. **In March 1931, another suit against Cornelius had been filed . . .** "Doctor's Clash with 'Naturopath': Evidence at Inquest," *The Herald* (Melbourne, Victoria, Australia), March 18, 1931. www.nla.gov.au.

17. **On trial, when asked if he had "taken any course of training" in regard to medicine, Cornelius responded that "practical experience on myself goes further" . . .** "Naturopath Questioned on His Fasting Theory," *The Herald* (Melbourne, Victoria, Australia), July 27, 1931. www.nla.gov.au.

18. **In what appear to be his booking photos taken February 1932 . . .** "41634 ROBERT De. V. Dreyer. Feb 1932 | Born Feb 1883," February 1932, National Archives of Australia: B741, V/11361, page 14, online.

19. **six-month stint in prison . . .** "6 Months for Naturopath: Dreyer Sentenced," The Herald (Melbourne, Victoria, Australia), November 5, 1931. www.nla.gov. au.

20. **Preached about his "false imprisonment" to a crowded hall of 300-400 people . . .** Copy of "BRIEF REPORT OF R. de VILLIER DREYER'S MEETING IN CENTRAL HALL ON 19.7.1933," July 19, 1933, National Archives of Australia: B741, V/11361, online.

21. **Won over a woman named Elva Mary Willing . . .** "Husband Has No Rights," *Truth* (Sydney, NSW, Australia), September 6, 1936. www.trove.nla. gov.au.

22. **Elva Mary had, what the couple deemed . . .** "World's Most Perfect Baby: Action in Court for Damages," *Truth* (Sydney, NSW, Australia), September 6, 1936. www.trove.nla.gov.au.

23. **Wahroonga Sanitarium had subjected Elva Mary . . .** "Baby Case: Libel Alleged," *The Sun* (Sydney, NSW, Australia), September 18, 1936. www.trove. nla.gov.au.

24. **"baby damnation" . . .** "Case Over Pamphlet on Babies," *The Labor Daily* (Sydney, NSW, Australia), September 19, 1936. www.trove.nla.gov.au.

25. **On September 28, 1936, it was reported . . .** "The Perfect Baby: Legal Dispute Sequel," *The Newcastle Sun* (Sydney, NSW, Australia), September 28, 1936. www.trove.nla.gov.au.

26. **"I could weep like Jesus for the destiny of mankind" . . .** Dreyer, *The Bible of Nature and the Book of Wisdom*, 81.

27. **Featuring entries in the index** . . . Dreyer, *The Bible of Nature and the Book of Wisdom*, V-X.
28. **Cornelius's face. In it, his thin lips are pursed** . . . Dreyer, *The Bible of Nature and the Book of Wisdom*, n.p.
29. **The more "poisons" you were loaded up with, the "uglier" you got** . . . Dreyer, *The Bible of Nature and the Book of Wisdom*, 155.
30. **"popular toxins"** . . . Dreyer, *The Bible of Nature and the Book of Wisdom*, 103.
31. **If you died ill and in pain, you deserved it; you had sinned** . . . Dreyer, *The Bible of Nature and the Book of Wisdom*, 34.
32. **("A natural man is a healthy man, and a healthy man is a moral man")** . . . Dreyer, *The Bible of Nature and the Book of Wisdom*, 101.
33. **If boys were allowed to partake in any food but what was "natural," they would cock their ears for "smutty yarn"** . . . Dreyer, *The Bible of Nature and the Book of Wisdom*, 88.
34. **"little trustful girls"** . . . Dreyer, *The Bible of Nature and the Book of Wisdom*, 85.
35. **"A beautiful girl of 18 years"** . . . Dreyer, *The Bible of Nature and the Book of Wisdom*, 55.
36. **"freshness" of "infantile" nineteen-year-olds** . . . Dreyer, *The Bible of Nature and the Book of Wisdom*, 209-210.
37. **"Fruitarians and other food faddists ascribe to fruit a health-giving potency which is entirely erroneous,"** . . . Dreyer, *The Bible of Nature and the Book of Wisdom*, 224.
38. **So, instead of fruit, in his book, he promised practitioners salvation** . . . Dreyer, *The Bible of Nature and the Book of Wisdom*, 226.
39. **In the late 1800s, refrigerated transport options meant that the price of meat lowered** . . . "Victorians: Food and Health," English Heritage. www.english-heritage.org.uk.
40. **In the early 1900s, World War I heightened these anxieties even further** . . . "A Picture of Health," National Portrait Gallery. www.npg.org.uk.
41. **In 1887, a woman named Pattie E. Beard** . . . Pattie E. Beard, "Good News for the Afflicted," *The Herald of the Golden Age*, United Kingdom: 69, 1897. www.google.com/books.
42. **HUGHES'S BLOOD PILLS!** . . . "Meddyginiaeth Rhyfeddaf Yr Oes!!" *Y Goleuad* (Wales), March 19, 1887. www.newspapers.library.wale.
43. **Seven long years of searching for a cure** . . . Pattie E. Beard, "Good News for the Afflicted," *The Herald of the Golden Age*, United Kingdom: 69, 1897. www.google.com/books.
44. **Beard, a stock broker, had hypnotized Pattie** . . . *Lucie Aldridge and Robjn Cantus, Before & After Great Bardfield: The Artistic Memoirs of Lucie Aldridge* (Inexpensive Progress, 2021), 16.
45. **Attended a lecture** . . . Pattie E. Beard, "Good News for the Afflicted," *The Herald of the Golden Age*, United Kingdom: 69, 1897. www.google.com/books.

46. **Wrote that she sold her bath chair after six months** . . . Pattie E. Beard, "Good News for the Afflicted," *The Herald of the Golden Age*, United Kingdom: 69, 1897. www.google.com/books.
47. **Finished their bowls of soup** . . . Lucie Aldridge and Robjn Cantus, *Before & After Great Bardfield*, 16-17.
48. ***The Beacon*** . . . Anna Wanigasekara, 'Research Question About the Beacon,' email, 2022.
49. **Sidney took visits from leaders in the vegetarian movement** . . . Charles W. Forward, *Fifty Years of Food Reform: A History of the Vegetarian Movement in England* (London: Ideal Publishing Union, 1898), 169.
50. **Backed by Sidney's financial power** . . . Aldridge and Cantus, *Before & After Great Bardfield*, 16.
51. **The Order of the Golden Age** . . . Forward, *Fifty Years of Food Reform*, 169.
52. **As Michelle Mary Lelwica writes** . . . Michelle Mary Lelwica, *Shameful Bodies: Religion and the Culture of Physical Improvement* (London: Bloomsbury Academic, an imprint of Bloomsbury Publishing, 2017), 25.
53. **In 1684, French physician François Bernier published "New Division of the Earth by the Different Species or Races of Man that Inhabit It,"** . . . Sabrina Strings, *Fearing the Black Body: The Racial Origins of Fat Phobia* (New York: New York University Press, 2019), 67.
54. **While once white women had been celebrated for their full figures** . . . Strings, *Fearing the Black Body*, 97-98.
55. **Religious leaders, physicians, and philosophers alike chimed in** . . . Strings, *Fearing the Black Body*, 97-99.
56. **George Cheyne** . . . R. S. Siddall, "George Cheyne, M.D.: Eighteenth Century Clinician and Medical Author," NCBI (1942), 98.
57. **Studying with Scottish physician Sir Archibald Pitcairne** . . . Westfall, Richard S., "Cheyne, George," *The Galileo Project*, Rice University, 2022. www.galileo.rice.edu.
58. **His friends in school were a group** . . . George Cheyne, *A Treatise on Health and Long Life* (London: W. Kidd, 1787), 184.
59. **and because of his time spent sedentary** . . . Strings, *Fearing the Black Body*, 100.
60. **A mirthful, kind, and humorous man by all written accounts** . . . Siddall, R.S., "George Cheyne, M.D.: Eighteenth Century Clinician and Medical Author," *Annals of Medical History*, 2022, 99. www.ncbi.nlm.nih.gov.
61. **Split his time "betwixt his patients and the punchbowl"** . . . Anne Charlton, "George Cheyne (1671 or 73-1743): 18th-century physician," *Journal of Medical Biography* 19 (2011): 50, DOI: 10.1258/jmb.2010.010028.
62. **He "grew excessively fat, short-breath'd, lethargic and listless"** . . . Anne Charlton, "George Cheyne (1671 or 73-1743): 18th-century physician," *Journal of Medical Biography* 19 (2011): 50, DOI: 10.1258/jmb.2010.010028.
63. **Rather than offer Cheyne aid** . . . George Cheyne, *Dr. Cheyne's Account of Himself and His Writings: Faithfully extracted from his various works* (J. Wilford, 1744), 2. www.books.google.com.

64. **Alone and unable to cure his own ailing body** . . . Anne Charlton, "George Cheyne (1671 or 73-1743): 18th-century physician," *Journal of Medical Biography* 19 (2011): 50, DOI: 10.1258/jmb.2010.010028.

65. **He recognized that he had been chasing "sensual Pleasures"** . . . Cheyne, Dr. Cheyne's Account of Himself and His Writings, 2. www.books.google.com.

66. **that a surprising cure was delivered to him by a fellow doctor** . . . Strings, *Fearing the Black Body*, 103.

67. **In his own words, he became "lank, fleet, and nimble,"** . . . Anne Charlton, "George Cheyne (1671 or 73-1743): 18th-century physician," *Journal of Medical Biography* 19 (2011): 50, DOI: 10.1258/jmb.2010.010028.

68. **as Strings writes, "a wide swath of haute English women."** . . . Strings, *Fearing the Black Body*, 116.

69. **One of these women, Lady Mary Wortley** . . . Strings, *Fearing the Black Body*, 115.

70. **While the milk diet ended up not working out** . . . Anne Charlton, "George Cheyne (1671 or 73-1743): 18th-century physician," *Journal of Medical Biography* 19 (2011): 50-51, DOI: 10.1258/jmb.2010.010028.

71. **he is not against "enlivening conversation, promoting friendship, comforting the sorrowful heart, and raising the drooping spirits by the cheerful cup"** . . . Anne Charlton, "George Cheyne (1671 or 73-1743): 18th-century physician," *Journal of Medical Biography* 19 (2011): 52, DOI: 10.1258/jmb.2010.010028.

72. **Sir Richard Phillips, in 1811, made a list of sixteen reasons to take up a vegetarian diet** . . . Howard Williams, *The Ethics of Diet: A Catena of Authorities Deprecatory of the Practice of Flesh-Eating* (London: F. Pitman, 1883), 240-241. www.archive.org.

73. **Others, like John Frank Newton, emphasized positive personal health benefits** . . . Williams, *The Ethics of Diet*, 206-207. www.archive.org.

74. **One man in particular who was influenced** . . . Williams, *The Ethics of Diet*, 259. www.archive.org.

75. **Cowherd made people sign an agreement promising to abstain from eating animals** . . . Williams, *The Ethics of Diet*, 259. www.archive.org.

76. **Though Cowherd passed in 1816** . . . Williams, *The Ethics of Diet*, 258. www.archive.org.

77. **In 1817, a group of two ministers, twenty adults, and nineteen children left England and endured an eleven-week journey** . . . Forward, *Fifty Years of Food Reform*, 13-15.

78. **On the morning of September 30, 1847** . . . Forward, *Fifty Years of Food Reform*, 22-24.

79. **In an excerpt from *Metamorphoses*** . . . John Smith, *Fruits and Farinacea: The Proper Food of Man, Being an Attempt to Prove, from History, Anatomy, Physiology, and Chemistry, that the Original, Natural, and Best Diet of Man is Derived from the Vegetable Kingdom* (New York: Fowler and Wells, 1854), 31.

80. **The Vegetarian Society split into two factions in 1888** . . . Margaret Puskar-Pasewicz, *Cultural Encyclopedia of Vegetarianism* (ABC-CLIO, 2010), 259.

81. **The Order of the Golden Age was founded in 1895** . . . John M. Gilheany, 2022, "The Order of the Golden Age: An Overview," *The Order of the Golden Age*. Accessed October 17, 2022. www.ordergoldenage.co.uk.

82. **While contemporarily the word "fruitarian"** . . . John M. Gilheany, 2022. "Fruitarian Society Feature," *The Order of the Golden Age*. Accessed October 17, 2022. www.ordergoldenage.co.uk.

83. **"When the Order of the Golden Age was founded** . . . John M. Gilheany, 2022, "The Order of the Golden Age: An Overview," *The Order of the Golden Age*. Accessed October 17, 2022. www.ordergoldenage.co.uk.

84. **"since about 1901, the Order of the Golden Age has come to the front"** . . . Samantha Calvert, "Eden's Diet: Christianity and Vegetarianism: 1809-2009," (PhD thesis, University of Birmingham, 2012), 214. www.etheses.bham.ac.uk.

85. **Convinced of the moral sanctity of their "fruitarianism,"** . . . Samantha Calvert, "Eden's Diet: Christianity and Vegetarianism: 1809-2009," (PhD thesis, University of Birmingham, 2012), 214. www.etheses.bham.ac.uk.

86. **"joints and tissues choked by waste and uric acid"** . . . Sidney H. Beard, "The Price of Physical Transgression," *The Herald of the Golden Age* 8, no. 2 (1910): 25.

87. **"the cause of a large proportion** . . . Sidney H. Beard, "Aims and Objects," *The Herald of the Golden Age* 16, (1913).

88. **In an article titled "Hygienic Christianity,"** . . . Sidney H. Beard, "Hygienic Christianity," *The Herald of the Golden Age* 7, no. 3 (1908): 41.

89. **"the great scientific fact** . . . Khursedji J. B. Wadia, "The Path of Purity," *The Herald of the Golden Age* 7, no. 2 (1908): 38.

Chapter 6: Guinea Pigs, Gurus, and People in Pain

1. **After about a month on the fruit diet** . . . Essie Honiball, *I Live on Fruit: Eat more fruit for a fruitful life* (South Africa: Essence of Health, 1981), 14-15.

2. **Cornelius most likely echoed advice he had communicated through his book** . . . Cornelius Valkenberg de Villiers Dreyer, *The Bible of Nature and the Book of Wisdom* (Sydney: "Dynamic Plus," 1936), 197.

3. **No alcohol, opium, whisky, tea, or coffee** . . . Dreyer, *The Bible of Nature and the Book of Wisdom*, 199.

4. **"sexual excesses and abuses."** . . . Dreyer, *The Bible of Nature and the Book of Wisdom*, 28.

5. **No frying food, for it destroys food value** . . . Dreyer, *The Bible of Nature and the Book of Wisdom*, 215.

6. **No high protein food** . . . Dreyer, *The Bible of Nature and the Book of Wisdom*, 53.

7. **. . . high protein foods are as sinful** . . . Dreyer, *The Bible of Nature and the Book of Wisdom*, 74.

8. **No insulin for diabetics, as it just poisons you further** . . . Dreyer, *The Bible of Nature and the Book of Wisdom*, 63.

9. **No prayer can make you purer;** . . . Dreyer, *The Bible of Nature and the Book of Wisdom*, 102.

10. **According to Dr. J. M. Good,** . . . Dreyer, *The Bible of Nature and the Book of Wisdom*, 41-42.

11. **Doctors are silly little pet Satans** . . . Dreyer, *The Bible of Nature and the Book of Wisdom*, 46.

12. **a field of alternative medical healers** . . . Dreyer, *The Bible of Nature and the Book of Wisdom*, 222, 226.

13. **In the late nineteenth century** . . . Susan E. Cayleff, *Nature's Path: A History of Naturopathic Healing in America* (Baltimore: Johns Hopkins University Press, 2016), 2.

14. **Alternative healers offered treatments** . . . Cayleff, *Nature's Path*, 4.

15. **Born in Michelbach, Germany** . . . Father Sebastian Kneipp . . . Cayleff, *Nature's Path*, 14, 28.

16. **He administered a series of "cold water" treatments to Lust** . . . Cayleff, *Nature's Path*, 28.

17. **Legend has it that after working with hygienic healer Dr. Sophie Scheel** . . . Cayleff, *Nature's Path*, 13.

18. **Women, vegetarians, religious devotees, spiritual and mental healers, and anti-vaccinationists** . . . Cayleff, *Nature's Path*, 2.

19. **Someone picking up an issue of** *The Herald of the Golden Age* . . . *The Herald of the Golden Age* 2, no. 10 (October 15, 1897): 122.

20. **In a criticism of experimentation on animals** . . . "Notes by the Way," *The Herald of the Golden Age* 2, no. 2 (November 13, 1897): 126.

21. **their rejection of evidence-based healing methods** . . . Cayleff, *Nature's Path*, 3.

22. **(As when Cornelius "Robert" Valkenberg de Villiers Dreyer** . . . "6 Months for Naturopath: Dreyer Sentenced," *The Herald* (Melbourne, Victoria, Australia), November 5, 1931. www.nla.gov.au.

23. **Mister Lust can make you well** . . . James C. Whorton, "Benedict Lust, Naturopathy, and the Theory of Therapeutic Universalism," *Iron Game History* 8, no. 2 (2003), 24.

24. **"morbid craving** . . . Christopher Hoolihan and Edward C. Atwater, *An Annotated Catalogue of the Edward C. Atwater Collection of American Popular Medicine and Health Reform, Volume 1* (Rochester: University of Rochester Press, 2001), 461.

25. **a litany of rules for how someone should carry out the treatment** . . . M.L. Holbrook, "The Grape Cure," *The Herald of the Golden Age* 2, no. 2 (1897): 125.

26. **In 1860, for example, Jean Charles Herpin** . . . Alice White, "The grape cure," Wellcome Collection, November 16, 2021. www.wellcomecollection.org.

27. **in 1927, a woman named Johanna Brandt set sail from her home** . . . Johanna Brandt, *The Grape Cure* (Summertown: Ehret Literature Publishing Company, 2014), 1-3.

28. **When Brandt turned forty** . . . Brandt, *The Grape Cure*, 5-10.

29. **After three months in New York City, Brandt** . . . Brandt, *The Grape Cure*, 3.

30. **Shackleton wrote about** . . . Basil Shackleton, *The Grape Cure: A Personal Testament* (Rochester: Thorsons Publishing Group, 1987), 10-15.

31. **Alcohol dependence that plagued him throughout his life** . . . Shackleton, *The Grape Cure,* 21, 24, 27, 28, 29, 30, 33.

32. **The warmth of a good woman was the only real cure for illness** . . . Shackleton, *The Grape Cure,* 37.

33. **Readers of the *Herald* would have seen** . . . R. A. De Rondan, "The Banana Cure," *The Herald of the Golden Age* 6, no. 1 (1901): 10.

34. **Monte Verità** . . . Arnold Ehret, *The Story of My Life* (New York: Benedict Lust Publications, 1980), 85-89.

35. **"The Value of the Banana,"** . . . "Value of the Banana," *The Herald of the Golden Age* 7, no. 8 (October 1909): 153.

36. **"The Banana Cure,"** . . . "The Banana Cure," *The Herald of the Golden Age* 6, no. 1 (January 15, 1901), 10.

37. **Josiah Oldfield** . . . Josiah Oldfield, "The Voice of Nature," *The Herald of the Golden Age* 7, no. 3 (July, 1908), 49.

38. **"confinement" brought about by industrialization** . . . William Earnshaw Cooper, "The Workman and His Food," *The Herald of the Golden Age* 7, no. 8 (July 1909), 144.

39. **Morris Krok, a South African** . . . O.L.M. Abramowski, *Fruitarian Diet & Physical Rejuvenation: A medical doctor's personal account of his health rejuvenation plan,* e-book: Living Nutrition, 2-3, 14. www.danmarkvaagner.dk.

40. **Brilliant stroke of isolated genius** . . . Honiball, *I Live on Fruit,* 12-13.

41. **Lisa Betty, a PhD candidate** . . . Lisa Betty, "Veganism* is in crisis," *Medium,* February 20, 2021. Accessed January 23, 2023. www.lbetty1.medium.com.

42. **As Khushbu Shah writes** . . . Khushbu Shah, "The Vegan Race Wars: How the Mainstream Ignores Vegans of Color," *Thrillist,* January 26, 2018. Accessed January 23, 2023. www.thrillist.com.

43. **PETA, according to Tara Roeder** . . . Lisa Betty, "Veganism* is in crisis," *Medium,* February 20, 2021. Accessed January 23, 2023. wwww.lbetty1.medium.com.

44. **As Amirah Mercer writes in her longform essay** . . . Amirah Mercer, "A Homecoming," *Eater,* January 14, 2021. Accessed January 23, 2023. www.eater.com.

45. **Isaias Hernandez, on his blog** . . . Hernandez, "Why Is There A Lack Of Diversity In Veganism?" *Queer Brown Vegan,* December 9, 2021. Accessed January 23, 2023. www.queerbrownvegan.com.

46. **Hernandez writes** . . . Isaias Hernandez, "What Is White Veganism?" *Queer Brown Vegan,* January 1, 2022. Accessed January 23, 2023. www.queerbrown-vegan.com.

47. **Sabrina Strings writes** . . . Sabrina Strings, *Fearing the Black Body: The Racial Origins of Fat Phobia* (New York: New York University Press, 2019), 6.

48. **They married and Essie writes** . . . Honiball, *I Live on Fruit,* 16.

49. **"no mercy"** . . . Honiball, *I Live on Fruit,* 12-13.

50. **Anoeschka von Meck, Essie's biographer** . . . Anoeschka von Meck (author, Essie Honiball's biographer), in discussion with the author. February 9, 2020 to June 14, 2022 via WhatsApp.

51. **Anoeschka told me about a moment so beautiful** . . . Anoeschka von Meck (author, Essie Honiball's biographer), in discussion with the author. February 9, 2020 to June 14, 2022 via WhatsApp.
52. **Not long after Cornelius whisked the two of them away in a van** . . . Anoeschka von Meck (author, Essie Honiball's biographer), in discussion with the author. February 9, 2020 to June 14, 2022 via WhatsApp.
53. **Essie spent each day sunning herself** . . . Honiball, *I Live on Fruit*, 16.

Chapter 7: Sick

1. **"Medicine can undermine our belief** . . . Susan Wendell, *The Rejected Body: Feminist Philosophical Reflections on Disability* (New York: Routledge, 1996), 122.
2. **"realities of bodily life"** . . . Wendell, *The Rejected Body*, 111.

Chapter 8: Testify

1. **God instructs Adam** . . . Genesis 2:15-17
2. **Scholars, when analyzing this moment in the text** . . . Bruce Wells, "Death in the Garden of Eden." *Journal of Biblical Literature* 1, December 2020; 139 (4): 639–660. DOI: https://doi.org/10.15699/jbl.1394.2020.1.
3. **When my browser first loaded** . . . Freelee, "30 Bananas a Day home page, February 28, 2012," *30 Bananas a Day*, www.web.archive.org.
4. **Fresh Dates!** . . . Freelee, "30 Bananas a Day homepage, February 16, 2012," *30 Bananas a Day*, www.web.archive.org.
5. **PK** . . . www.web.archive.org.
6. **Freelee and Durianrider called it** . . . "A Vision," *30 Bananas a Day*, February 18, 2012. www.web.archive.org.
7. **Members joined from Sweden** . . . "All Members," *30 Bananas a Day*, www. web.archive.org.
8. **one member was "brought here by** . . . "anna bruce." *The Frugivore Diet*, website now deleted. www.thefrugivorediet.com.
9. **"fight his stage 4 lung cancer"** . . ."Kerstin Jessup," *The Frugivore Diet*, www. thefrugivorediet.com.
10. **One member, Raini Pachak** . . . Raini Pachak (former member of 30BaD), in discussion with the author. June 15, 2020 via Zoom.
11. **In his profile picture on the site** . . . Raini Pachak. *The Frugivore Diet*, website now deleted. www.thefrugivorediet.com.
12. **"I met cool people on *30 Bananas a day*,"** . . . Raini Pachak (former member of 30BaD), in discussion with the author. June 15, 2020 via Zoom.
13. **"Frequently Asked Questions"** . . . "Frequently Asked Questions," *30 Bananas a Day*, www.web.archive.org.
14. **the page's header featured** . . . "Testify!" *30 Bananas a Day*, www.web. archive.org.
15. **Comment by Shannana Bannana** . . . Shannana Bannana, "Comment on Testify!" *30 Bananas a Day*, July 3, 2011. www.web.archive.org.

16. **My skin is clear! I'm rarely bloated!** . . . "Ashley Christensen <3" posted April 23, 2011, "melissa jackson," October 7, 2010: "Comments on Testify!" *30 Bananas a Day,* www.web.archive.org.

17. **When Freelee posted a montage video** . . . Freelee The Banana Girl, "Freelee banana girl before and after vegan lifestyle," YouTube Video, 4:17, August 29, 2011. www.youtube.com.

18. **No cheat days, no sick days** . . . PK, "30BaD Banana Wagon Tour," December 8, 2011. www.web.archive.org.

Chapter 9: Finding the Fruit

1. **Search "Freelee and Durianrider"** . . . Cid Dwyer, "Freelee & Durianrider: The Most DANGEROUS Vegan Couple," YouTube Video, 34:38, July 31, 2022. www.youtube.com.

2. **or "Freelee The Banana Girl and Durianrider** . . . Tom Lauris, "Freelee The Banana Girl and Durianrider: Eating Disorders For Life," YouTube Video, 19:31, December 13, 2022. www.youtube.com.

3. **(a *Daily Mail* article** . . . Daniel Piotrowski and Emily Crane, "I could retire in 100 countries on the money I earn pimping my girlfriend out": Sleazy boast by boyfriend of Banana Girl lifestyle guru revealed in legal battle with Bikini Girl," *Daily Mail,* March 26, 2015. www.dailymail.co.uk.

4. **2016 *Jezebel* piece in which Ellie Shechet** . . . Ellie Shechet, "A Year of Bananas, Vasectomies, and Rape Allegations With the Vegans of YouTube," *Jezebel,* November 2, 2016. www.jezebel.com.

5. **"Monkey business,"** . . . Abby Haglage, "Why the '30 Bananas a Day Diet' Is Monkey Business," *Daily Beast,* January 2, 2014 (updated July 12, 2017). www.thedailybeast.com.

6. **"bananas," and "insane."** . . . Tess Koman, "This Insane Instagram Diet Involves Eating 30 Bananas a Day," *Cosmopolitan,* September 16, 2014. www.cosmopolitan.com.

7. **"Cosmo Mag calls my diet INSANE!!"** . . . Freelee The Banana Girl, "Cosmo Mag calls my diet INSANE!! My response on Banana Island," YouTube Video, 8:20, September 17, 2014. www.youtube.com.

8. **28,130 people had created accounts on the site** . . . "All Members (28,130)," *30 Bananas a Day,* April 9, 2015. www.web.archive.org.

9. **382,923 subscribed to Freelee's YouTube Account** . . . "Freelee the Banana Girl," YouTube Channel, June 30, 2015. www.web.archive.org.

10. **Following rose to 789,311 by July 2019** . . . "Freelee The Banana Girl," YouTube Channel, July 11, 2019. www.web.archive.org.

11. **Just 9,823 people were using the site** . . . "All Members (9,823)," *30 Bananas a Day,* March 12, 2012. www.web.archive.org.

12. **Freelee was sharing tips like** . . . "Freelee's Top 10 Tips for Health," *Fruit-Powered: Natural Health Services, Media & Store,* May 1, 2013. www.fruit-powered.com.

13. **"Sure, I'd be happy to chat."** Durianrider, "Interview Request," email, 2023.

14. **"Author, International speaker and educator** . . . Freelee The Banana Girl, *Go Fruit Yourself: How I Lost 40 LBS on a Raw Food Lifestyle & Regained My Health* (Self-published), 3.

15. **was a child who was raised on a farm** . . . Freelee, *Go Fruit Yourself,* 6.

16. **stripped from their mothers and being "permanently confined** . . . Freelee, *Go Fruit Yourself,* 90-91.

17. **"Rip the calf away from her nipple,"** . . . Freelee, *Go Fruit Yourself,* 92.

18. **Teeth were "raped" of their innocence** . . . Freelee, *Go Fruit Yourself,* 80.

19. **Leanne was only allowed a couple pieces** . . . Freelee, *Go Fruit Yourself,* 6.

20. **Athletic performances** . . ."Your thoughts on Durianrider? Dude ran a 2:48 thon off 10 miles a week," *LetsRun,* January 28, 2018. www.letsrun.com.

21. **Public persona** . . . "What do you really think of durianrider?" *Reddit,* 2015. www.reddit.com.

22. **"The Ugly Truth About Harley 'Durianrider' Johnstone"** "The Ugly Truth About Harley 'Durianrider' Johnstone," *Anthony Colpo,* March 3, 2016, www. anthonycolpo.com.

23. **"A Year of Bananas, Vasectomies, and Rape Allegations With the Vegans of YouTube"** Ellie Shechet, "A Year of Bananas, Vasectomies, and Rape Allegations with the Vegans of YouTube," *Jezebel,* November 4, 2016. Accessed August 17, 2022. www.jezebel.com.

24. **There is a video of his current girlfriend** . . . Harley Johnstone (@durianrider_). 2023. "What 178 cm @61kg looks like. The best investment a girl can make is doing my protocols so she enhances/preserves her life freedom, health, aesthetics, relationships, hormones, finances and mental/physical performance." Instagram Photo, January 14, 2023. www.instagram.com.

25. **In another, his girlfriend is wearing a white crop top** . . . Harley Johnstone (@durianrider_). 2023. "Next time you get told carbs are fattening ALWAYS remember us and how slim we are FEASTING every day. MOST cyclists are fat. MOST runners are fat. Just go watch any marathon or Gran Fonda and you will see MOST of the entries are fat. So much for 'oh but you exercise that's why you are slim'. Natasha at 178cm and 61.7kg Pic from friday night. Natasha bought my ebook when she was 17 and had never restricted her refined sugar intake in her life. She has gotten better with age which is VERY rare from 17-24 because most girls get told and sold lies that make them fat or STRUGGLE to keep a BMI under 20. Just look around. It's very very sad. ZERO women want legs that rub together or arms that look like ham hocks or a caffeine addiction that ages them RAPIDLY for the worse. My protocols GUARANTEE you will get a strip-per body! GUARANTEED!! You will also feel your best mentally. You will feel better in hours." Instagram Photo, December 3, 2022. www.instagram.com.

26. **"HTFU. If you don't know what this means. Google it."** . . . Harley Johnstone, *Carb the Fuck Up: Follow Your Heart With No Fucks Given* (Self-published), 99.

27. **Tumblr, when asked, "Can you cite any successes as a cyclist or runner,"** . . . Durianrider, "Can you cite any successes as a cyclist or runner?" Tumblr, 2021. www.askdurianrider.tumblr.com.

28. **Harley Johnstone, at the age of eight** . . . Johnstone, *Carb the Fuck Up*, 11.

29. **"chronic fatigue, asthma, Crohn's disease** . . . "80/10/10 Allstar: Harley Johnstone: Ultra Endurance Mountain Bike Champion," *FoodnSport*, December 11, 2009. www.foodnsport.com.

30. **"light and delicate** . . . Johnstone, *Carb the Fuck Up*, 11.

31. **I can envision him crooning gently** . . . Harley Johnstone (@durianrider_). Instagram post now deleted.

32. **Comparing his ex-girlfriend to Amber Heard** . . . Harley Johnstone (@durianrider_). "FL has been slandering me daily for 6 years. Her similarities to Ambuser Heard are startling. Who she is on camera isn't who she is IRL. Who spins their BS better to get their audience to give them sympathy? I'd give that prize to FL hands down because she spreads rumours behind the scenes and stays silent when those rumours get wildly exaggerated. Robin's best hope now is to jump on the back of Casey the Cassowary and hightail out of Cape Tribulation whilst he can. No wonder he looks so stressed these days. I imagine he would stay up late at night looking at the mosquitos getting eaten by the geckos on the ceiling and thinking what his future holds after seeing what she has done me. As a man you are guilty until proven innocent. Screenshots are better than any lawyer. Make sure you have them Robin." Instagram Photo, July 14, 2022. www.instagram.com.

33. **Fat-shaming Calvin Klein models** . . . Harley Johnstone (@durianrider_). "I made my boy Vegan Gains so famous he and his lady got scalped by CK" Instagram Photo, September 11, 2022. www.instagram.com.

34. **Spreading conspiracy theories about COVID-19** . . . Harley Johnstone (@durianrider_). "Looonk at these hippies crying about put a jab. I'm sure it's safe! According to the FDA 108 days is enough testing time to give a new drug to anyone and everyone. Roll up your sleeves and do what the government and mainstream media (who represent the trillion dollar brands) direct you to do. Don't question what they encourage. This is for your health! You want to be healthy right?" Instagram Photo, March 6, 2022. www.instagram.com.

35. **At sixteen, Leanne left her family's farm** . . . Freelee, *Go Fruit Yourself*, 6.

36. **"graveyard for innocent tortured animals."** . . . Freelee The Banana Girl, *The Raw Till 4 Diet: Banana Girl Cleanse* (Self-published), 8.

37. **"a male calf in a veal crate** . . . Freelee The Banana Girl, *My Naked Lunchbox: The Most Controversial Cookbook Ever Written* (Self-published), 18.

38. **She took up swimming** . . . Freelee, *My Naked Lunchbox*, 19-20.

39. **Leanne soon realized he was a drug dealer** . . . Freelee, *Go Fruit Yourself*, 7.

40. **working her job at the supermarket** . . . Freelee, *My Naked Lunchbox*, 20.

41. **"Yeh bitches you just jealous."** . . . Freelee, *The Raw Till 4 Diet*, 8.

42. **After four or so years** . . . Freelee, *The Raw Till 4 Diet*, 8.

43. **Leanne broke up with her then-boyfriend** . . . Freelee, *Go Fruit Yourself*, 8.

44. **She got breast implants** . . . Freelee, *My Naked Lunchbox*, 191-192.

45. **"resembled a Barbie doll"** Freelee, *My Naked Lunchbox*, 191.

46. **"worthy, and validated"** Freelee, *My Naked Lunchbox*, 192.

47. **Harley left his childhood home** . . . Johnstone, *Carb the Fuck Up*, 151-152.

48. **"didn't even know what the word gratitude meant back then"** Johnstone, *Carb the Fuck Up*, 153-154.
49. **"I instantly regretted it"** . . . Johnstone, *Carb the Fuck Up*, 152.
50. **At her lowest** . . . Freelee, *Go Fruit Yourself*, 8-9.
51. **Tired of pills** . . . Freelee, *The Raw Till 4 Diet*, 10.
52. **It was then, in 2006** . . . Freelee, *Go Fruit Yourself*, 9.
53. **He finds a bush turkey** . . . Johnstone, *Carb the Fuck Up*, 153-154.

Chapter 10: Banana Island

1. **In 2007, she read books like *Raw Food Detox Diet*** . . . Freelee The Banana Girl, *The Raw Till 4 Diet: Banana Girl Cleanse* (Self-published), 8.
2. **"Are We Herbivores?"** . . . Douglas N. Graham, The 80/10/10 Diet: Balancing Your Health, Your Weight, and Your Life, One Lucious Bite at a Time (U.S.: FoodnSport Education, 2010), 24-29.
3. **Almost invariably,"** . . . Graham, *The 80/10/10 Diet*, 102.
4. **"Humans vs. Carnivores** . . . Graham, *The 80/10/10 Diet*, 17-20.
5. **John Smith published a book** . . . John Smith, *Substance Of The Work Entitled Fruits And Farinacea, The Proper Food Of Man* (London: The Vegetarian Society's Depot, 1880), 14-16.
6. **"It's not a new idea under the sun."** Douglas Graham (creator of 80/10/10 diet), Zoom with author, May 28, 2023.
7. **had his own blog.** Doug Graham, "FoodNSport.com: Defining the Cause of Health." www.foodnsport.com.
8. **In one of them, Graham sits beside one of his practitioners** . . . GameTastic, "BANANA ISLAND Explained by Dr. Douglas N Graham," 5:22. www.web. archive.org.
9. **A raw vegan named Liz** . . . Liz Bunting. "Why Banana Island?" *The Raw Herbalist*, April 21, 2017. Accessed January 16, 2023. www.therawherbalist.com.
10. **In his interview with MC Fructose** . . . "BANANA ISLAND Explained by Dr. Douglas N Graham," 5:22. www.web.archive.org.
11. **Leanne, after attending the picnic** . . . Freelee, The Raw Till 4 Diet, 10-11.
12. **Author Victoria Moran boarded a Greyhound bus** . . . "Natural Hygiene 1990: The Straight and Narrow Never Looked So Good!" *Vegetarian Times*, no. 153 (May 1991): 56-60.
13. **Natural Hygiene, an offshoot of naturopathy** . . . Susan E. Cayleff, *Nature's Path: A History of Naturopathic Healing in America* (Baltimore: Johns Hopkins University Press, 2016), 29.
14. **Graham's fascination with wellness** . . . Mildred V. Naylor, "Sylvester Graham, 1794-1851." *Annals of Medical History*, vol. 4 (3) (May 1942): 236-240. www.ncbi.nlm.nih.gov.
15. **William Alcott was publishing prolifically** . . . Cayleff, *Nature's Path*, 30.
16. **"vegetarianism, sunlight, frequent bathing** . . . Cayleff, *Nature's Path*, 30.
17. **"opening bedroom windows** . . . "Natural Hygiene 1990: The Straight and Narrow Never Looked So Good!" *Vegetarian Times*, no. 153 (May 1991): 56-60.

18. **natural hygiene was reintroduced . . .** "Natural Hygiene 1990: The Straight and Narrow Never Looked So Good!" *Vegetarian Times*, no. 153 (May 1991): 56-60.

19. **"matter" that "came before the Board of Chiropractic."** Board of Chiropractic vs. Douglas N. Graham, 97-005960 (Marathon, FL. 1998).

20. **"These people were not patients."** Douglas Graham (creator of 80/10/10 diet), Zoom with author, May 28, 2023.

21. **a twenty-five-year-old woman . . .** Board of Chiropractic vs. Douglas N. Graham, 97-005960 (Marathon, FL. 1998).

22. **"Yeah, I knew a fair bit about Tim."** Douglas Graham (creator of 80/10/10 diet), Zoom with author, May 28, 2023.

23. **"he had not done any examination that would permit him to appropriately treat K.E."** Board of Chiropractic vs. Douglas N. Graham, 97-005960 (Marathon, FL. 1998).

24. **"she thought that some kind of relationship was going to happen that never did. She got very upset and so she turned her vengeance on me."** Douglas Graham (creator of 80/10/10 diet), Zoom with author, May 28, 2023.

25. **K.E.'s weight dropped to a dangerously low 87 pounds . . .** Board of Chiropractic vs. Douglas N. Graham, 97-005960 (Marathon, FL. 1998).

26. **"eventually, under oath,"** Douglas Graham (creator of 80/10/10 diet), Zoom with author, May 28, 2023.

27. **described dabbling in vegetarianism . . .** Douglas Graham (creator of 80/10/10 diet), Zoom with author, May 28, 2023.

28. **"hygienic (nutritionally sound) lifestyle based on . . .** Board of Chiropractic vs. Douglas N. Graham, 97-005960 (Marathon, FL. 1998).

29. **Doctor of Chiropractic from Life Chiropractic College . . .** Douglas Graham (creator of 80/10/10 diet), Zoom with author, May 28, 2023.

30. **"The degree was bestowed a long time ago."** Doug Graham, "Follow-up Questions," email, 2023.

31. **"They never came to my office" . . .** Douglas Graham (creator of 80/10/10 diet), Zoom with author, May 28, 2023.

32. **Brian arrived at Club Hygiene on November 7, 1993 . . .** Board of Chiropractic vs. Douglas N. Graham, 97-005960 (Marathon, FL. 1998).

33. **"We did not discuss HIV six years prior."** Douglas Graham (creator of 80/10/10 diet), Zoom with author, May 28, 2023.

34. **"rejected as inherently improbable and unworthy of belief."** Board of Chiropractic vs. Douglas N. Graham, 97-005960 (Marathon, FL. 1998).

35. **"anal infection, frequent diarrhea, weight loss . . .** Board of Chiropractic vs. Douglas N. Graham, 97-005960 (Marathon, FL. 1998).

36. **"No. I can't tell you where that idea came from . . .** Douglas Graham (creator of 80/10/10 diet), Zoom with author, May 28, 2023.

37. **B.D. drank only water for nine days . . .** Board of Chiropractic vs. Douglas N. Graham, 97-005960 (Marathon, FL. 1998).

38. **"He weighed himself."** Douglas Graham (creator of 80/10/10 diet), Zoom with author, May 28, 2023.

39. **Brian began eating solid food.** Board of Chiropractic vs. Douglas N. Graham, 97-005960 (Marathon, FL. 1998).

40. **"Within hours of his coming, maybe a day . . .** Douglas Graham (creator of 80/10/10 diet), Zoom with author, May 28, 2023.

41. **On December 7, 1993, someone called an ambulance . . .** Board of Chiropractic vs. Douglas N. Graham, 97-005960 (Marathon, FL. 1998).

42. **Graham's license to practice as a chiropractor was . . .** Board of Chiropractic vs. Douglas N. Graham, 97-005960 (Marathon, FL. 1998).

43. **"paperwork monitored for six months."** Douglas Graham (creator of 80/10/10 diet), Zoom with author, May 28, 2023.

44. **In 2011, on an online message board . . .** Nzreva, "Going to Health fest for 3 days," *The Project Avalon Forum: Chronicles of the human awakening,* November 27, 2013. www.projectavalon.net.

45. **"Yes, she had a heart problem and died in the hospital" . . .** Douglas Graham (creator of 80/10/10 diet), Zoom with author, May 28, 2023.

46. **"When I graduated from Life Chiropractic College . . ."** Doug Graham, "Follow-up Questions," email, 2023.

47. **In January 2014, after paying the $8,000 entry fee, Leah Hodge . . .** Leah Hodge, "Nearly died on 25 Day Water Fast with Doug Graham," YouTube video, 26:44, August 13, 2014. www.youtube.com.

48. **"Sure. Fasting is inappropriate for a phenomenal number of people . . ."** Douglas Graham (creator of 80/10/10 diet), Zoom with author, May 28, 2023.

49. **"fit, healthy and well just plain awesome!" . . .** Freelee, *The Raw Till 4 Diet,* 11.

50. **One night, for example, she visited two different sushi places . . .** Freelee The Banana Girl, *Go Fruit Yourself: How I Lost 40 LBS on a Raw Food Lifestyle & Regained My Health* (Self-published), 10.

51. **"To be frank," she writes, "it was fucking soul destroying." . . .** Freelee, *The Raw Till 4 Diet,* 11.

52. **A Tony Robbins seminar saved her . . .** Freelee, *Go Fruit Yourself,* 10.

53. **They went out to an open-air market together . . .** Durianrider, "Freelee The Banana Girl Before I Made Her Viral," YouTube video, 0:32, December 5, 2008. www.youtube.com.

54. **After spending more and more time together . . .** Freelee, *Go Fruit Yourself,* 10.

55. **"I remember when I first met Freelee . . .** Durianrider, "How I knew Freelee was the girl for me," YouTube video, 3:55, July 24, 2015. www.youtube.com.

56. **They started dating . . .** Freelee, *Go Fruit Yourself,* 11.

57. **"Hi, my name is Freelee," . . .** Freelee The BananaGirl, "Why I eat a low fat raw vegan diet," YouTube video, 4:51, January 4, 2009. www.youtube.com.

Chapter 11: The Fruititionist

1. **Freelee's offer of two thirty-minute Skype calls . . .** Freelee, "FREELEE." *30 Bananas a Day,* February 14, 2012. Accessed January 17, 2023 through WayBack Machine. www.web.archive.org.

2. **Freelee and Durianrider caricatured . . .** "30 Bananas a Day: The High Carb Raw Vegan Lifestyle," *30 Bananas a Day*, February 14, 2012. Accessed January 17, 2023 through WayBack Machine. www.web.archive.org.

3. **the "steam room" . . .** Freelee, "Please keep all swearing to the 'Steam Room,'" *30 Bananas a Day*, February 14, 2012. Accessed January 17, 2023 through WayBack Machine. www.web.archive.org.

4. **(like "How often should I eliminate?" . . .** The Phenomenal Lauren G, "How often should I eliminate?" *30 Bananas a Day*, February 8, 2012. Accessed January 17, 2023 through WayBack Machine. www.web.archive.org.

5. **His first, aptly titled . . .** Durianrider, "Durianrider First Ever Youtube Video June 23rd 2008 #retro," YouTube video, 0:09, June 24, 2008. www.youtube. com.

6. **The second video he ever posted . . .** Durianrider, "Durianrider: Blood and bones or fruit and veg? #2," YouTube video, 0:19, June 24, 2008. www.youtube. com.

7. **In them, he films himself yet again at the market . . .** Durianrider, "primal diet is for freaks..#11," YouTube video, 0:39, July 5, 2008. www.youtube.com.

8. **In a different clip, he explains his moniker . . .** Durianrider, "why they call me durianrider #4," YouTube video, 0:11, June 26, 2008. www.youtube.com.

9. **In another, with a yellow and green Specialized helmet . . .** Durianrider, "durianrider: primal diet is for sickos!," YouTube video, 1:06, October 9, 2008. www.youtube.com.

10. **His personal blog, DURIANRIDER'S BLOG, . . .** "DURIANRIDER'S BLOG." Accessed via Wayback Machine. www.web.archive.org.

11. **I talked with . . .** James and Dahlia Marin (RDNs, CEO, and CEO of Married to Health), Zoom with author, February 10, 2023.

12. **I remember the era . . .** 53meal, "Freelees Weight loss on raw food Q &," YouTube video, 10:09, April 23, 2012. www.youtube.com.

13. **In one of her first, she says hello to the camera . . .** Freelee The Banana Girl, "How much fruit I eat in a day on Go Fruit Yourself," YouTube video, 3:12, September 18, 2011. www.youtube.com.

14. **Christine (Davidsson) Sandal, in her thesis . . .** Christine Sandal, "You are what you eat online: The phenomenon of mediated eating practices and their underlying moral regimes in Swedish 'What I eat in a day' vlogs" (Master's thesis, Lund University, May 2018). www.lup.lub.lu.se.

15. *Refinery29* **credits . . .** Amelia Tate, "TikTok's 'What I Eat in a Day' & Our Obsession With What Other People Eat," *Refinery 29*, June 21, 2021. www. refinery29.com.

16. **In Essie Honiball's memoir . . .** Essie Honiball, *I Live on Fruit: Eat more fruit for a fruitful life* (South Africa: Essence of Health, 1981), 21-31.

17. **Arnold Ehret, the one who claimed that fasting and fruit healed him . . .** Arnold Ehret, *Professor Arnold Ehret's Mucusless Diet Healing System: Scientific Method of Eating Your Way to Health* (Summertown, TN: Ehret Literature Publishing Company, 2013), 85, 88.

18. **"living cesspool" . . .** Ehret, *Mucusless Diet Healing System*, 50.

19. **"worms and decades-old feces-stones"** . . . Ehret, *Mucusless Diet Healing System*, 18.
20. **the "unknown, decayed and fermented mass of matter** . . . Ehret, *Mucusless Diet Healing System*, 125.
21. **He started selling a laxative called "INNER-CLEAN,"** . . . Arthur J. Cramp, *Nostrums and Quackery and Pseudomedicine*, vol. 3 (Chicago: American Medical Association, 1936), 72. www.babel.hathitrust.org.
22. **Even as of 2020, there is a Facebook group** . . . Pro Spira, "Welcome to the Mucusless Diet Support Group! (Please Read)," Facebook Group, May 28, 2020. Accessed January 17, 2023. www.facebook.com.
23. **Historically, as Christine Sandal notes in her thesis** . . . Sandal, "You are what you eat online," 20.
24. **acknowledged the origins of veganism** . . . Sabrina Strings, *Fearing the Black Body: The Racial Origins of Fat Phobia* (New York: New York University Press, 2019), 118.
25. **As Sandal notes, vlogging daily eats is a mashup** . . . Sandal, "You are what you eat online," 17.
26. **Unlike in the past** . . . Sandal, "You are what you eat online," 21.
27. **Freelee's emphasis on clean eating** . . . Lauren Coleman (former follower of Freelee), in discussion with the author. September 27, 2020 via Zoom.
28. **Brandt claimed that grapes** . . . Johanna Brandt, *The Grape Cure* (Summertown: Ehret Literature Publishing Company, 2014), 46.
29. **Ehret, in his Mucusless Diet Healing System** . . . Ehret, *Mucusless Diet Healing System,* 12.
30. **"filthy, mostly constipated colon** . . . Ehret, *Mucusless Diet Healing System*, 112.
31. **Madonna-like, holy purity"** . . . Ehret, *Mucusless Diet Healing System*, 114.
32. **As for Essie, she says that Cornelius** . . . Honiball, *I Live on Fruit*, 42.
33. **she remembers fainting two or three** . . . Honiball, *I Live on Fruit*, 13.
34. **Cornelius took a fall** . . . Anoeschka von Meck (author, Essie Honiball's biographer), in discussion with the author. February 9, 2020 to June 14, 2022 via WhatsApp.
35. **Before he passed, he told Essie to stay true to fruit. His last words to her were, "See How far you can go and how high you can aim."** . . . Honiball, *I Live on Fruit*, 40-41.
36. **Essie tried her best to stay on the right path** . . . Honiball, *I Live on Fruit*, 12.
37. **She attended dinner parties** . . . Anoeschka von Meck (author, Essie Honiball's biographer), in discussion with the author. February 9, 2020 to June 14, 2022 via WhatsApp.
38. **Friends, scientists, and doctors alike** . . . Honiball, *I Live on Fruit*, 12, 18.
39. **In her memoir she writes** . . . Honiball, *I Live on Fruit*, 38-39.
40. **Early in her fruit journey, Freelee was scared** . . . Freelee The Banana Girl, "Day 10: Why sometimes eating cooked food is BETTER than RAW FOOD," YouTube video, 6:24, June 10, 2013. www.youtube.com.

Chapter 12: Salvation, Starvation

1.   **At the time I was watching, in 2012 . . .** "Freelee TV: The Raw Fit Bitch,"
     YouTube Channel. Accessed via WayBack Machine. www.web.archive.org.
2.   **In a video, "How to become a SLAVE to the system," . . .** Freelee The Banana
     Girl, "How to become a SLAVE to the system.(funny)," YouTube video, 5:39,
     December 27, 2011. www.youtube.com.
3.   **As Christine Sandal writes . . .** Christine Sandal, "You are what you eat online:
     The phenomenon of mediated eating practices and their underlying moral re-
     gimes in Swedish 'What I eat in a day' vlogs" (Master's thesis, Lund University,
     May 2018), 56. www.lup.lub.lu.se.
4.   **In her videos, often while wearing a cropped green "Go Fruit Yourself"
     T-shirt . . .** Freelee The Banana Girl, "Bananas ONLY diet! I ate bananas only
     for weeks," YouTube video, September 28, 2011. www.youtube.com.
5.   **"Anorexia is brought about by poor nutrition . . .** Freelee The Banana Girl,
     *Go Fruit Yourself: How I Lost 40 LBS on a Raw Food Lifestyle & Regained My
     Health* (Self-published), 21-23.
6.   **By Freelee's fifth video posted to YouTube . . .** Freelee The Banana Girl,
     "RAW FOOD WEIGHT LOSS: I eat up to 50 bananas a day!" YouTube video,
     9:57, April 22, 2010. www.youtube.com.
7.   **One member of 30BaD, Paden Janney . . .** "Paden Janney," *The Frugivore Diet.*
     Accessed January 17, 2023. Website now deleted. www.thefrugivorediet.com.
8.   **On October 7, 2012 . . .** Paden Janney, "Starting my 30 Day Challenge," *30
     Bananas a Day*, October 7, 2012. Accessed January 23, 2023 via WayBack
     Machine. www.web.archive.org.
9.   **In a 2018 Reddit thread posted under r/EDAnonymous . . .** u/crashdiet-
     dummy, "Fuck freelee the banana girl," Reddit. Accessed January 23, 2023.
     www.reddit.com.
10. **In a 2018 article "Strict health-oriented eating patterns . . .** Anna Brytek-
     Matera, Kamila Czepczor-Bernat, Helena Jurzak, Monika Kornack, and Natalia
     Kolodziejcyk, "Strict health-oriented eating patterns (orthorexic eating behav-
     iours) and their connection with a vegetarian and vegan diet," *Eating and Weight
     Disorders 24*, no. 3 (August 2018). www.ncbi.nlm.nih.gov.
11. **Some of them gathered on an eating disorder forum . . .** "banana girl diet,
     raw fit bitch, high carb vegan diet, freelee the banana girl." *ED Support Forum.*
     www.edsupportforum.com.
12. **"I came from a lot of family struggles," . . .** (anonymous former follower), in
     discussion with the author. April 10, 2020 via phone call.

Chapter 13: Rebuke the Unclean Spirit

1.   **In the seventh century BCE, a man was confined to his bed for observa-
     tion . . .** Troels Pank Arbøll, "A Newly Discovered Drawing of a Neo-Assyrian
     Demon in BAM 202 Connected to Psychological and Neurological Disorders,"
     Le Journal des Medecines Cuneiformes, no. 33 (2019): 4. www.academia.edu.
2.   **The creature was a physical representation of *bennu* . . .** Troels Pank
     Arbøll, "A Newly Discovered Drawing of a Neo-Assyrian Demon in BAM

202 Connected to Psychological and Neurological Disorders," *Le Journal des Medecines Cuneiformes*, no. 33 (2019): 6. www.academia.edu.

3. **In ancient Mesopotamia . . .** Theresa Machemer, "This Demon, Immortalized in 2,700-Year-Old Assyrian Tablet, Was Thought to Cause Epilepsy," *Smithsonian Magazine*, January 3, 2020. www.smithsonianmag.com.

4. **In the village of Slätthög in Småland, Sweden . . .** Mia Tuft and Karl O. Nakken, "Epilepsy as stigma – evil, holy or mad?" www.tidsskriftet.no/en.

5. **"You unbelieving and perverse generation," . . .** Matthew 17:17.

6. **"This meant progress and gave me courage for what lay ahead . . .** Essie Honiball, *I Live on Fruit: Eat more fruit for a fruitful life* (South Africa: Essence of Health, 1981), 15.

Chapter 14: Pints of Milk and Boiled Potatoes (Fruit Yourself! Root Yourself!)

1. **Titled "How to start a RAW FOOD / Raw till 4 Diet today!" . . .** Freelee The Banana Girl, "How to start a RAW FOOD / Raw till 4 Diet today!" YouTube video, 10:16, June 5, 2012. www.youtube.com.

2. **Like Durianrider's 2009 . . .** Durianrider, "RAW FOOD VEGAN FALLS OFF THE COOKED FOOD WAGON! #91," YouTube video, 2:07, December 11, 2009. www.youtube.com.

3. **"Freelee the Fruititionist's" posts . . .** Freelee The Banana Girl, "Frequently Asked Questions," *30 Bananas a Day*, September 30, 2009. Accessed January 18, 2023 via WayBack Machine. www.web.archive.org.

4. **In November 2011, when Freelee posted an eleven-minute video . . .** Freelee The Banana Girl, "Freelee's top 10 tips to stay FullyRaw and get rid of cooked food cravings," YouTube video, 11:06, November 8, 2011. www.youtube.com.

5. **Later in the Raw Till 4 Introduction video . . .** Freelee The Banana Girl, "How to start a RAW FOOD / Raw till 4 Diet today!" YouTube video, 10:16, June 5, 2012. www.youtube.com.

6. **"adopted a partly raw lifestyle"** Freelee The Banana Girl, "How RT4 Was Born," *The Raw Till 4 Diet: Banana Girl Cleanse*, 32.

7. **"potatoes, root veggies, rice, gluten-free pasta," . . .** "What is the Raw Till 4 Diet?" *The Banana Girl*. www.thebananagirl.com.

8. **"a specific event or was there a realization over time" . . .** Brian Rossiter, "Harley Johnstone on the Woodstock Fruit Festival Controversy, Changing Focus," *Fruit-Powered*, December 5, 2013. www.fruit-powered.com.

9. **claimed to thrive for a time . . .** Arnold Ehret, *The Story of My Life* (New York: Benedict Lust Publications, 1980), 98, 117.

10. **stick to fresh fruit, raw celery, lettuce . . .** Arnold Ehret, *Professor Arnold Ehret's Mucusless Diet Healing System: Scientific Method of Eating Your Way to Health* (Summertown, TN: Ehret Literature Publishing Company, 2013), 75.

11. **Essie Honiball once got a craving for milk . . .** Anoeschka von Meck (author, Essie Honiball's biographer), in discussion with the author. February 9, 2020 to June 14, 2022 via WhatsApp.

12. **"Oh, you probably don't mind** ... Essie Honiball, *I Live on Fruit: Eat more fruit for a fruitful life* (South Africa: Essence of Health, 1981), 39.

13. **Anoeschka described the symptoms** ... Anoeschka von Meck (author, Essie Honiball's biographer), in discussion with the author. February 9, 2020 to June 14, 2022 via WhatsApp.

14. **She lists out the sly way in which she transitioned a man who loved** ... Honiball, *I Live on Fruit,* 58-62.

15. **A bunch of fruitarians head to Camp Walden** ... "Tentative Schedule 2012." *The Woodstock Fruit Festival.* Accessed January 18, 2023 via WayBack Machine. www.web.archive.org.

16. **Freelee and Durianrider, alongside founder Michael Arnstein** ... "The Pioneers 2012," *The Woodstock Fruit Festival.* Accessed January 18, 2023 via WayBack Machine. www.web.archive.org.

17. **which means they were compensated for their attendance** ... Alexandra Kleeman, "This means raw: extreme dieting and the battle among fruitarians," *The Guardian,* December 3, 2010. www.theguardian.com.

18. **The board of governors (including Graham)** ... Michael Arnstein, "Harley and Freelee, No Longer Pioneers; Now Speical Guests," *The Woodstock Fruit Festival,* November 23, 2013. Accessed January 18, 2023 via WayBack Machine. www.web.archive.org.

19. **In the video, posted December 2, 2013** ... Freelee The Banana Girl, "Kicked off as pioneers at Woodstock Fruit Festival, our reaction," YouTube video, 16:40, December 2, 2013. www.youtube.com.

20. **"I've been Fully Raw, Raw Till 4** ... LITWAI, "HENYA MANIA Banned From Rawtill4 Thai Fruit Festival!?!" YouTube video, 4:27, March 28, 2016. www.youtube.com.

21. **"I've always promoted eating whatever you wanna eat** ... Henya Mania, Facebook post. www.facebook.com.

22. **Durianrider took umbrage with the fact** ... Durianrider, "FREELEE BANNED ME FOR LYING! Response," YouTube video, 11:02, March 25, 2016. www.youtube.com.

23. **In one, a user named LITWAI** ... LITWAI, "HENYA MANIA Banned From Rawtill4 Thai Fruit Festival!?!" YouTube video, 4:27, March 28, 2016. www.youtube.com.

24. **An example is a post by a 30BaD user** ... ag, "Something feels wrong. Too wrong. Need some advice. Please!" *30 Bananas a Day,* March 29, 2013. Accessed January 18, 2023 via WayBack Machine. www.web.archive.org.

Chapter 15: The Serpent Tricked Me

1. **"We want to make the garden bigger for everyone,"** ... Freelee The Banana Girl, "Kicked off as pioneers at Woodstock Fruit Festival, our reaction," YouTube video, 16:40, December 2, 2013. www.youtube.com.

2. **(Official Music Video)" begins with an address** ... Petit Reklaitis, "Raw Till 4 Thai Fruit Festival (Official Music Video)," YouTube video, 6:21, September 5, 2015. www.youtube.com.

3. **In one video, Freelee adds twenty dates to a blender** . . . Freelee the Banana Girl, "What I ate today on a high carb diet," YouTube video, 5:28, July 24, 2013. www.youtube.com.

4. **English Toffee Sweet Drops®** . . . "English Toffee Sweet Drops ®, 288 Servings," *SweetLeaf,* 2022. Accessed August 15, 2022. www.sweetleaf.com/.

5. **Though Freelee clarified to her "glucose junkies"** . . . Freelee The Banana Girl, "Day 19: RAW TILL 4 DIET VS FULLYRAW DIET," YouTube video, 8:32, June 19, 2013. www.youtube.com.

6. **She started eating heaping bowls of corn pasta** . . . Freelee The Banana Girl, "Time lapse of me eating a 1700cal bowl of pasta," YouTube video, 6:38, October 23, 2013. www.youtube.com.

7. **went to what appears to be a mall food court for plates** . . . Durianrider, "What I Eat In A Day 100% Day 4," YouTube video, 9:52, November 9, 2013. www.youtube.com.

8. **One of these was the transformation of someone** . . . Fat2FitonFRUIT, "Fat 2 Fit on FRUIT – My transformation story," YouTube video, 7:14, December 11, 2013. www.youtube.com.

9. **When someone on Snapchat asked** . . . Anna Kaiye, "RT4 left me Broke, Fat, and Unhappy," YouTube video, 11:37, July 15, 2016. www.youtube.com.

10. **One such person was Anna** . . . Anna Kaiye, (Tried the 80/10/10 high-carb, low-fat, raw vegan diet for nearly two years), in discussion with the author. July 6, 2020 via Zoom.

11. **Instead, she recorded herself trying on clothes** . . . Anna Kaiye, "RT4 left me Broke, Fat, and Unhappy," YouTube video, 11:37, July 15, 2016. www. youtube.com.

12. **After consuming such massive quantities of fruit** . . . Anna Kaiye, (Tried the 80/10/10 high-carb, low-fat, raw vegan diet for nearly two years), in discussion with the author. July 6, 2020 via Zoom.

13. **I asked James and Dahlia Marin, the two plant-based dieticians** . . . James and Dahlia Marin (RDNs, CEO, and CEO of Married to Health), in discussion with the author. February 10, 2023 via Zoom.

14. **In her e-book** *The Raw Till 4 Diet* . . . Freelee The Banana Girl, "How RT4 Was Born," *The Raw Till 4 Diet: Banana Girl Cleanse,* 36, 37, 38.

15. **"I was laying the groundwork before it got better,"** . . . Anna Kaiye, (Tried the 80/10/10 high-carb, low-fat, raw vegan diet for nearly two years), in discussion with the author. July 6, 2020 via Zoom.

16. **Instead, on day one of the festival** . . . Javier S., "Opening Raw Till 4 Thai Fruit Festival 2015 Durianrider & Freelee The Banana Girl," YouTube video, 45:43, July 9, 2015. www.youtube.com.

17. **Anna describes having "an echo chamber in that community"** . . . Anna Kaiye, (Tried the 80/10/10 high-carb, low-fat, raw vegan diet for nearly two years), in discussion with the author. July 6, 2020 via Zoom.

18. **The former follower who wishes to remain anonymous** . . . (anonymous former follower), in discussion with the author. April 10, 2020 via phone call.

19. **In the video of their welcome Q&A event by the pond** . . . Javier S., "Opening Raw Till 4 Thai Fruit Festival 2015 Durianrider & Freelee The Banana Girl," YouTube video, 45:43, July 9, 2015. www.youtube.com.

20. **choreographed flash dance in the park** . . . Freelee The Banana Girl, "Undercarbed low energy boring people at the Thai Fruit Festival :(," YouTube video, 4:44. June 11, 2015. www.youtube.com.

21. **As Freelee explains in a video** . . . Freelee The Banana Girl, "Thai Fruit Fest Drama My thoughts and Review," YouTube video, 7:02, June 27, 2015. www. youtube.com.

22. **Durianrider says, "[Man]** . . . **immature, inexperienced, spoiled brat."** . . . Martha Minch Mccrate, "Annie Jaffery & Jil VS Joe Best The saga finally ending," YouTube video, 16:28, August 7, 2015. www.youtube.com.

23. **He made videos like "HOT babe with flat stomach gets negged by Durianrider"** . . . Durianrider, "HOT babe with flat stomach gets negged by Durianrider," YouTube video, 0:57, July 19, 2012. www.youtube.com.

24. **He posted a video where he filmed Freelee** . . . Durianrider, "Hot sexy fitness model parades for 130lb skinny vegan boyfriend," YouTube video, 3:13, October 9, 2012. www.youtube.com.

25. **"We look at the big picture** . . . Freelee The Banana Girl, "Thai Fruit Fest Drama My thoughts and Review," YouTube video, 7:02, June 27, 2015. www. youtube.com.

26. **Instead, as revealed in an interview for a *Jezebel* article** . . . Ellie Shechet, "A Year of Bananas, Vasectomies, and Rape Allegations with the Vegans of YouTube," *Jezebel,* November 4, 2016. Accessed August 17, 2022. www.jezebel. com.

27. **to Freelee blaming a person's death from cancer** . . . Freelee The Banana Girl, "Youtube celebrity passes on," YouTube video, 11:47, July 26, 2013. www. youtube.com.

28. **"When your obese brothers and sisters get stuck on the stairwell** . . . Danny Gold, "Is This The Worst Person On The Internet?" *Gawker,* February 27, 2012. Accessed January 18, 2023. www.gawker.com.

29. **In the comments on her video "Why did Selena Gomez gain weight?** . . . Freelee The Banana Girl, "Why did Selena Gomez gain weight? Call me girlfriend!," YouTube video, June 6, 2015. www.youtube.com.

Chapter 16: A Different Kind of Garden

1. **Back at the first farm gathering in Cairns** . . . Freelee The Banana Girl, "Rawfood Vegan Retreat in Australia!" YouTube video, 9:58, December 13, 2009. www.youtube.com.

2. **But when I look back on the videos that they posted in 2009** . . . Durianrider, "Freelee The Banana Girl Before I Made Her Viral," YouTube video, 0:32, December 5, 2008. www.youtube.com.

3. **I see Durianrider at the market** . . . Durianrider, "primal diet is for freaks..#11," YouTube video, 0:39, July 5, 2008. www.youtube.com.

4. **I see grainy footage of produce laid out on a rug . . .** Freelee The Banana Girl, "How much fruit I eat in a day on Go Fruit Yourself," YouTube video, 3:12, September 18, 2011. www.youtube.com.

5. **"carbed-up soldiers" . . .** Durianrider, "Ethics & Goals of RT4 Thai Fruit Festival," YouTube video, 1:47, July 20, 2014. www.youtube.com.

6. **In one video, breaking open the carefully curated image . . .** Durianrider, "FREELEE EATING IN PRIVATE BUSTED ON CAMERA!" YouTube video, 0:50, February 3, 2016. www.youtube.com.

7. **In another, Durianrider revealed just how far he had fallen . . .** Durianrider, "100% What I Ate Today Day 32," YouTube video, 2:42, March 28, 2016. www.youtube.com.

8. **"That first year we had was the Thai Fruit Festival . . .** Durianrider, "Raw Till 4 Thai Bike Festival Rules," YouTube video, 8:38, March 24, 2016. www.youtube.com.

9. **They purged their group of all the "drainbows" . . .** Plantriotic, "RAW TILL 4 BIKE FEST BANNED (RESPONSE)," YouTube video, 7:19, March 27, 2016. www.youtube.com.

10. **Lex, who preferred jiu-jitsu to cycling . . .** Lex, "I'm a Shit Cunt | Thai Fruit Fest Drama | Ask DurianRider Myself," YouTube video, 5:28, May 9, 2016. www.youtube.com.

11. **The candy-coated version of the Raw Till 4 Festival . . .** Bonny Rebecca, "FIRST DAY IN THAILAND // VEGAN DINNER + RIDING MOUNTAINS," YouTube video, 10:29, June 4, 2016. www.youtube.com.

12. **On the last day of the Raw Till 4 Festival . . .** Durianrider, "Answering questions for 2 hours on camera," YouTube video, 1:49:43, June 22, 2016. www.youtube.com.

13. **In 2015, Durianrider made a video saying Freelee . . .** HighCarbWeightLoss, "How much money does Freelee / Freelala make? Per month?!" YouTube video, 2:51, March 19, 2015. www.youtube.com.

14. **In 2022, he claimed she has made "millions and millions" . . .** Durianrider, "Freelee The Banana Girl & Why Im Suing Her For 3 Million," 10:39, July 15, 2022. www.youtube.com.

15. **Durianrider says, "We'll still be hanging around during the week . . .** Durianrider, "Answering questions for 2 hours on camera," YouTube video, 1:49:43, June 22, 2016. www.youtube.com.

16. **In September 2016, Freelee and Durianrider publicly announced . . .** Durianrider, "Freelee The Banana Girl & Why I Broke It Off With Her," YouTube video, 13:20, September 16, 2016. www.youtube.com.

17. *Jezebel* **reported that a former follower . . .** Ellie Shechet, "A Year of Bananas, Vasectomies, and Rape Allegations with the Vegans of YouTube," *Jezebel,* November 4, 2016. Accessed August 17, 2022. www.jezebel.com.

18. **(Freelee, on Tumblr, later posted she did . . .** "Raw Vegan RawTill4," Tumblr. www.rawjola.tumblr.com.

19. **Freelee accused Durianrider of using steroids . . .** Daniel Peters, "'If you hit like a man you're going to get hit back': Ex-partner of Vegan vlogger Freelee the

Banana Girl says she was 'manipulative, violent and secretly using botox.'" *Daily Mail,* September 28, 2016. www.dailymail.co.uk.

20. **The former follower who wishes to remain anonymous, who had wholly embraced the tenants of the lifestyle** . . . (anonymous former follower), in discussion with the author. April 10, 2020 via phone call.

21. **video Freelee created in response to Anna's "Raw Till 4 (RT4) left me Fat, Broke, & Unhappy"** . . . *The Frugivore Diet,* "Freelee reacts to Raw Till 4 (RT4) left me Fat, Broke & Unhappy (the truth) #70," YouTube video, 35:32, May 6, 2021. www.youtube.com

22. **Durianrider, who had once felt like "a brother, of sorts"** . . . Happy Healthy Vegan, "Durianrider: Apologize . . ." YouTube video, 7:05, December 6, 2016. www.youtube.com.

23. **"It's almost like I was dreaming or acting,"** . . . (anonymous former follower) in discussion with the author. April 10, 2020 via phone call.

24. **"a supermajority of Doug's peers** . . . "Secondary Information Document In the matter of Doug Graham and his relationship to the Woodstock Fruit Festival." www.docs.google.com.

25. **"a mutual thing"** . . . Douglas Graham (creator of 80/10/10 diet), Zoom with author, May 28, 2023.

26. **"I was dropped as a pioneer** . . . Doug Graham, "Follow-up Questions," email, 2023.

27. **A Level 1 certification is available for $997** . . . "The 80/10/10 Coaching Certification," www.811coach.com.

28. **Prices that range from $7,500 to $9,000** . . . "Detoxification, Cleansing, and Healing in Costa Rica," *FoodnSport.* www.foodnsport.com.

29. **"I've never wanted a bigger piece of the pie"** . . . Douglas Graham (creator of 80/10/10 diet), Zoom with author, May 28, 2023.

30. **Durianrider lives in Australia now** . . . Askdurianrider, Tumblr, "I lived in cairns for 6 months in summer . . ." January 2023. www.tmblr.co.

31. **He cycles** . . . Durianrider, "Cycling Australia Adelaide Style," YouTube Shorts, February 8, 2023. www.youtube.com.

32. **Has a fondness toward spiders** . . . Durianrider, "This spider needs your help," YouTube Shorts, December 28, 2022. www.youtube.com.

33. **Remains a high-carb vegan** . . . Durianrider, "How To Get To 4% Body Fat The RIGHT Way," YouTube video, March 16, 2023. www.youtube.com.

34. **believes that copious amounts of cane sugar added to each meal are necessary** . . . Durianrider, "Sugar & The Bitter Truth With Durianrider," YouTube video, 46:07, May 12, 2019. www.youtube.com.

35. **He has denied all allegations of sexual assault** . . . Ellie Shechet, "A Year of Bananas, Vasectomies, and Rape Allegations With the Vegans of YouTube," *Jezebel,* November 2, 2016. www.jezebel.com.

36. **currently dating a woman named Natasha** . . . Zaczek, "Vegan cyclist YouTuber who used to go out with Freelee the Banana Girl is bashed in front of his new girlfriend at a market," *Daily Mail,* January 18, 2020. www.dailymail. co.uk.

37. **"If Her Back Doesn't Need Adjusting, She Isn't The Right Girl For You,"** Durianrider, "If Her Back Doesn't Need Adjusting, She Isn't The Right Girl For You," YouTube video, 3:25, September 1, 2022. www.youtube.com.

38. **"How much money should you spend on women so they respect you?"** . . . Durianrider, "How much money should you spend on women so they respect you?" YouTube video, 35:04, August 23, 2022. www.youtube.com.

39. **In one video titled "The Truth About Her Body** . . . Durianrider, "The Truth About Her Body & Cycling Shoes WILL Shock You," YouTube video, 4:25, August 9, 2022. www.youtube.com.

40. **"dystopian future"** . . . Freelee The Banana Girl, "4 months of freedom left? Why you must leave the city now," YouTube video, 13:44, September 3, 2020. www.youtube.com.

41. **She left Australia for Ecuador** . . . Freelee The Banana Girl, "Off Grid, Jungle Life and Food Forest with Freelee," YouTube Playlist. www.youtube.com.

42. **In 2018, she authored a feminist manifesto of sorts** . . . Freelee The Banana Girl, *My Naked Lunchbox: The Most Controversial Cookbook Ever Written* (Self-published), 191.

43. **"What I eat in a day in recovery"** . . . *The Frugivore Diet*, "What I eat in a day in recovery," YouTube video, 12:17, April 30, 2023. www.youtube.com.

Chapter 17: How to Heal

1. **After meeting T.O. Honiball, she still found herself floundering** . . . Anoeschka von Meck (author, Essie Honiball's biographer), in discussion with the author. February 9, 2020 to June 14, 2022 via WhatsApp.

2. **"Was I being vegan because I said I was vegan** . . . (anonymous former follower), in discussion with the author. April 10, 2020 via phone call.

3. **Lauren Coleman, the person who once carted giant banana smoothies to her job** . . . Lauren Coleman (former follower of Freelee), in discussion with the author. September 27, 2020 via Zoom.

4. **There was Raini Pachak, the teenager from Utah** . . . Raini Pachak (former member of 30BaD), in discussion with the author. June 15, 2020 via Zoom.

5. **There was Bonny Rebecca** . . . Bonny Rebecca, "Why I'm no longer vegan . . ." YouTube video, 38:04, January 14, 2019. www.youtube.com.

6. **There was Anna** . . . Anna Kaiye, (tried the 80/10/10 high-carb, low-fat, raw vegan diet for nearly two years), in discussion with the author. July 6, 2020 via Zoom.

7. **"As long as there was any trace of hatred** . . . Essie Honiball, *I Live on Fruit: Eat more fruit for a fruitful life* (South Africa: Essence of Health, 1981), 93.